**WHO guidelines
for indoor air quality:
dampness and mould**

Keywords

AIR POLLUTION, INDOOR - adverse effects - prevention and control
FUNGI
HUMIDITY - adverse effects - prevention and control
ENVIRONMENTAL EXPOSURE
RISK ASSESSMENT
GUIDELINES

ISBN 798 92 890 4168 3

Address requests for publications of the WHO Regional Office for Europe to:
    Publications
    WHO Regional Office for Europe
    Scherfigsvej 8
    DK-2100 Copenhagen Ø, Denmark
Alternatively, complete an online request form for documentation, health information, or for permission to quote or translate, on the Regional Office web site (http://www.euro.who.int/pubrequest).

Edited by: Elisabeth Heseltine and Jerome Rosen.
Cover photos (from top): © Heger/Müller, © Szewzyk, © UBA, picture taken by Moriske.
Book design: Sven Lund.
Printed in Germany by Druckpartner Moser.

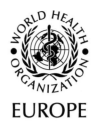

EUROPE

WHO guidelines for indoor air quality: dampness and mould

Abstract

Microbial pollution is a key element of indoor air pollution. It is caused by hundreds of species of bacteria and fungi, in particular filamentous fungi (mould), growing indoors when sufficient moisture is available. This document provides a comprehensive review of the scientific evidence on health problems associated with building moisture and biological agents. The review concludes that the most important effects are increased prevalences of respiratory symptoms, allergies and asthma as well as perturbation of the immunological system. The document also summarizes the available information on the conditions that determine the presence of mould and measures to control their growth indoors. WHO guidelines for protecting public health are formulated on the basis of the review. The most important means for avoiding adverse health effects is the prevention (or minimization) of persistent dampness and microbial growth on interior surfaces and in building structures.

Contents

Contributors

Participants in the working group meeting in Bonn, 17–18 October 2007

Alireza Afshari	Danish Building Research Institute, Copenhagen, Denmark
Hugh Ross Anderson[1]	St George's Hospital Medical School, University of London, London, England
Aaron Cohen[1]	Health Effects Institute, Boston, United States of America
Eduardo de Oliveira Fernandes	Institute of Mechanical Engineering, Faculty of Engineering, University of Porto, Porto, Portugal
Jeroen Douwes	Centre for Public Health Research, Massey University, Wellington, New Zealand
Rafal Górny	Institute of Occupational Medicine and Environmental Health, Sosnowiec, Poland
Maija-Riitta Hirvonen	National Public Health Institute, Helsinki, Finland
Jouni Jaakkola	Institute of Occupational and Environmental Medicine, University of Birmingham, Birmingham, United Kingdom
Séverine Kirchner[1]	Centre Scientifique et Technique du Bâtiment, Marne la Vallée France
Jarek Kurnitski	University of Technology, Helsinki, Finland
Hal Levin	Building Ecology Research Group, Santa Cruz, United States of America
Mark Mendell	Lawrence Berkeley National Laboratory, Berkeley, United States of America
Lars Mølhave[1]	Department of Public Health, University of Aarhus, Aarhus, Denmark
Lidia Morawska	International Laboratory for Air Quality and Health, Queensland University of Technology, Brisbane, Australia
Aino Nevalainen[1]	National Public Health Institute, Helsinki, Finland

Malcolm Richardson	University of Helsinki, Helsinki, Finland
Peter Rudnai	National Institute of Environmental Health, Budapest, Hungary
Hans W. Schleibinger	Institute for Research in Construction, National Research Council of Canada, Ottawa, Canada
Per E. Schwarze	Norwegian Institute of Public Health, Oslo, Norway
Bernd Seifert[1]	Consultant, Berlin, Germany
Torben Sigsgaard	University of Aarhus, Aarhus, Denmark
Weimin Song	Fudan University, Shanghai, China
John Spengler[1]	Harvard School of Public Health, Boston, United States of America
Regine Szewzyk	Federal Environment Agency, Berlin, Germany
Sadras Panchatcharam Thyagarajan	Sri Ramachandra University, Chennai, India
Giulio Gallo	European Commission, Brussels, Belgium
Manfred Giersig (observer)	European Chemical Industry Council (CEFIC) and Bayer Material Science AG, Leverkusen, Germany

Co-authors who did not participate in the working group meeting

Jakob Bønløkke	University of Aarhus, Aarhus, Denmark
Kerry Cheung	Centre for Public Health Research, Massey University, Wellington, New Zealand
Anna G. Mirer	Lawrence Berkeley National Laboratory, Berkeley, United States of America
Harald W. Meyer	Hillerød Hospital, Hillerød, Denmark
Marjut Roponen	National Public Health Institute, Helsinki, Finland

[1] Steering Group member

Reviewers who did not participating in the working group meeting

Olaf Adan   Eindhoven University of Technology and
                                    Netherlands Organization for Applied Scientific
                                    Research (TNO), Eindhoven, Netherlands

Gwang Pyo Ko   Seoul National University, Seoul,
                                    Republic of Korea

WHO Regional Office for Europe

Matthias Braubach

Otto Hänninen

Michal Krzyzanowski (project leader)

Secretariat: Andrea Rhein, Deepika Sachdeva

None of the people listed declared any conflict of interest.

Acknowledgements

Preparation of the guidelines was supported by funds received by the WHO European Centre for Environment and Health (Bonn Office) from the German Federal Environment Ministry and from the United Kingdom Department of Health, which are gratefully acknowledged.

The input of Jeroen Douwes was supported by a Sir Charles Hercus Fellowship funded by the Health Research Council of New Zealand.

Foreword

Healthy indoor air is recognized as a basic right. People spend a large part of their time each day indoors: in homes, offices, schools, health care facilities, or other private or public buildings. The quality of the air they breathe in those buildings is an important determinant of their health and well-being. The inadequate control of indoor air quality therefore creates a considerable health burden.

Indoor air pollution – such as from dampness and mould, chemicals and other biological agents – is a major cause of morbidity and mortality worldwide. About 1.5 million deaths each year are associated with the indoor combustion of solid fuels, the majority of which occur among women and children in low-income countries.

Knowledge of indoor air quality, its health significance and the factors that cause poor quality are key to enabling action by relevant stakeholders – including building owners, developers, users and occupants – to maintain clean indoor air. Many of these actions are beyond the power of the individual building user and must be taken by public authorities through the relevant regulatory measures concerning building design, construction and materials, and through adequate housing and occupancy policies. The criteria for what constitutes healthy indoor air quality provided by these guidelines are therefore essential to prevent disease related to indoor air pollution.

These guidelines were developed by the WHO Regional Office for Europe in collaboration with WHO headquarters as part of the WHO programme on indoor air pollution. Further guidelines on indoor air quality in relation to pollution emanating from specific chemicals and combustion products are under development.

The *WHO guidelines on indoor air quality: dampness and mould* offer guidance to public health and other authorities planning or formulating regulations, action and policies to increase safety and ensure healthy conditions of buildings. The guidelines were developed and peer reviewed by scientists from all over the world, and the recommendations provided were informed by a rigorous review of all currently available scientific knowledge on this subject. We at WHO thank these experts for their efforts, and believe that this work will contribute to improving the health of people around the world.

Marc Danzon
WHO Regional Director for Europe

Executive summary

This document presents World Health Organization (WHO) guidelines for the protection of public health from health risks due to dampness, associated microbial growth and contamination of indoor spaces. The guidelines are based on a comprehensive review and evaluation of the accumulated scientific evidence by a multidisciplinary group of experts studying health effects of indoor air pollutants as well as those specialized in identification of the factors that contribute to microbial growth indoors.

Problems of indoor air quality are recognized as important risk factors for human health in both low-income and middle- and high-income countries. Indoor air is also important because populations spend a substantial fraction of time within buildings. In residences, day-care centres, retirement homes and other special environments, indoor air pollution affects population groups that are particularly vulnerable due to their health status or age. Microbial pollution involves hundreds of species of bacteria and fungi that grow indoors when sufficient moisture is available. Exposure to microbial contaminants is clinically associated with respiratory symptoms, allergies, asthma and immunological reactions.

The microbial indoor air pollutants of relevance to health are widely heterogeneous, ranging from pollen and spores of plants coming mainly from outdoors, to bacteria, fungi, algae and some protozoa emitted outdoors or indoors. They also include a wide variety of microbes and allergens that spread from person to person. There is strong evidence regarding the hazards posed by several biological agents that pollute indoor air; however, the WHO working group convened in October 2006 concluded that the individual species of microbes and other biological agents that are responsible for health effects cannot be identified. This is due to the fact that people are often exposed to multiple agents simultaneously, to complexities in accurately estimating exposure and to the large numbers of symptoms and health outcomes due to exposure. The exceptions include some common allergies, which can be attributed to specific agents, such as house-dust mites and pets.

The presence of many biological agents in the indoor environment is due to dampness and inadequate ventilation. Excess moisture on almost all indoor materials leads to growth of microbes, such as mould, fungi and bacteria, which subsequently emit spores, cells, fragments and volatile organic compounds into indoor air. Moreover, dampness initiates chemical or biological degradation of materials, which also pollutes indoor air. Dampness has therefore been suggested to be a strong, consistent indicator of risk of asthma and respiratory symptoms (e.g. cough and wheeze). The health risks of biological contaminants of indoor air could thus be addressed by considering dampness as the risk indicator.

Health hazards result from a complex chain of events that link penetration of water indoors, excessive moisture to biological growth, physical and chemical degradation, and emission of hazardous biological and chemical agents. The review of scientific evidence that supports these guidelines follows this sequence of events. The issues related to building dampness and its effect on indoor exposure to biological and non-biological pollutants are summarized in Chapter 2, which also addresses approaches to exposure assessment. An important determinant of dampness and biological growth in indoor spaces is ventilation, and this issue is discussed in Chapter 3. The evidence for the health effects of indoor exposure is presented in Chapter 4, based on a review of epidemiological studies and of clinical and toxicological research on the health effects of dampness and mould. The results of the epidemiological and toxicological studies are summarized in the appendices.

The background material for the review was prepared by invited experts and discussed at a WHO working group meeting, convened in Bonn, Germany, 17–18 October 2007. The conclusions of the working group discussion are presented in Chapter 5 and are reproduced in this executive summary, as follows.

- Sufficient epidemiological evidence is available from studies conducted in different countries and under different climatic conditions to show that the occupants of damp or mouldy buildings, both houses and public buildings, are at increased risk of respiratory symptoms, respiratory infections and exacerbation of asthma. Some evidence suggests increased risks of allergic rhinitis and asthma. Although few intervention studies were available, their results show that remediation of dampness can reduce adverse health outcomes.
- There is clinical evidence that exposure to mould and other dampness-related microbial agents increases the risks of rare conditions, such as hypersensitivity pneumonitis, allergic alveolitis, chronic rhinosinusitis and allergic fungal sinusitis.
- Toxicological evidence obtained in vivo and in vitro supports these findings, showing the occurrence of diverse inflammatory and toxic responses after exposure to microorganisms isolated from damp buildings, including their spores, metabolites and components.
- While groups such as atopic and allergic people are particularly susceptible to biological and chemical agents in damp indoor environments, adverse health effects have also been found in nonatopic populations.
- The increasing prevalences of asthma and allergies in many countries increase the number of people susceptible to the effects of dampness and mould in buildings.

The conditions that contribute to the health risk were summarized as follows.

- The prevalence of indoor dampness varies widely within and among countries, continents and climate zones. It is estimated to affect 10–50% of indoor environments in Europe, North America, Australia, India and Japan. In certain settings, such as river valleys and coastal areas, the conditions of dampness are substantially more severe than the national averages for such conditions.
- The amount of water on or in materials is the most important trigger of the growth of microorganisms, including fungi, actinomycetes and other bacteria.
- Microorganisms are ubiquitous. Microbes propagate rapidly wherever water is available. The dust and dirt normally present in most indoor spaces provide sufficient nutrients to support extensive microbial growth. While mould can grow on all materials, selection of appropriate materials can prevent dirt accumulation, moisture penetration and mould growth.
- Microbial growth may result in greater numbers of spores, cell fragments, allergens, mycotoxins, endotoxins, β-glucans and volatile organic compounds in indoor air. The causative agents of adverse health effects have not been identified conclusively, but an excess level of any of these agents in the indoor environment is a potential health hazard.
- Microbial interactions and moisture-related physical and chemical emissions from building materials may also play a role in dampness-related health effects.
- Building standards and regulations with regard to comfort and health do not sufficiently emphasize requirements for preventing and controlling excess moisture and dampness.
- Apart from its entry during occasional events (such as water leaks, heavy rain and flooding), most moisture enters a building in incoming air, including that infiltrating through the building envelope or that resulting from the occupants' activities.
- Allowing surfaces to become cooler than the surrounding air may result in unwanted condensation. Thermal bridges (such as metal window frames), inadequate insulation and unplanned air pathways, or cold water plumbing and cool parts of air-conditioning units can result in surface temperatures below the dew point of the air and in dampness.

On the basis of this review, the following guidelines were formulated.

- Persistent dampness and microbial growth on interior surfaces and in building structures should be avoided or minimized, as they may lead to adverse health effects.
- Indicators of dampness and microbial growth include the presence of condensation on surfaces or in structures, visible mould, perceived mouldy odour

and a history of water damage, leakage or penetration. Thorough inspection and, if necessary, appropriate measurements can be used to confirm indoor moisture and microbial growth.

- As the relations between dampness, microbial exposure and health effects cannot be quantified precisely, no quantitative health-based guideline values or thresholds can be recommended for acceptable levels of contamination with microorganisms. Instead, it is recommended that dampness and mould-related problems be prevented. When they occur, they should be remediated because they increase the risk of hazardous exposure to microbes and chemicals.

- Well-designed, well-constructed, well-maintained building envelopes are critical to the prevention and control of excess moisture and microbial growth, as they prevent thermal bridges and the entry of liquid or vapour-phase water. Management of moisture requires proper control of temperatures and ventilation to avoid excess humidity, condensation on surfaces and excess moisture in materials. Ventilation should be distributed effectively throughout spaces, and stagnant air zones should be avoided.

- Building owners are responsible for providing a healthy workplace or living environment free of excess moisture and mould, by ensuring proper building construction and maintenance. The occupants are responsible for managing the use of water, heating, ventilation and appliances in a manner that does not lead to dampness and mould growth. Local recommendations for different climatic regions should be updated to control dampness-mediated microbial growth in buildings and to ensure desirable indoor air quality.

- Dampness and mould may be particularly prevalent in poorly maintained housing for low-income people. Remediation of the conditions that lead to adverse exposure should be given priority to prevent an additional contribution to poor health in populations who are already living with an increased burden of disease.

The guidelines are intended for worldwide use, to protect public health under various environmental, social and economic conditions, and to support the achievement of optimal indoor air quality. They focus on building characteristics that prevent the occurrence of adverse health effects associated with dampness or mould. The guidelines pertain to various levels of economic development and different climates, cover all relevant population groups and propose feasible approaches for reducing health risks due to dampness and microbial contamination. Both private and public buildings (e.g. offices and nursing homes) are covered, as dampness and mould are risks everywhere. Settings in which there are particular production processes and hospitals with high-risk patients or sources of exposure to pathogens are not, however, considered.

While the guidelines provide objectives for indoor air quality management, they do not give instructions for achieving those objectives. The necessary action and indicators depend on local technical conditions, the level of development, human capacities and resources. The guidelines recommended by WHO acknowledge this heterogeneity. In formulating policy targets, governments should consider their local circumstances and select actions that will ensure achievement of their health objectives most effectively.

1. Introduction

1.1 Background

Problems of indoor air quality are recognized as important risk factors for human health in both low-income and middle- and high-income countries. Indoor air is important also because populations spend a substantial fraction of time within buildings. In residences, day-care centres, retirement homes and other special environments, indoor air pollution affects population groups that are particularly vulnerable due to their health status or age. Microbial pollution involves hundreds of species of bacteria and fungi that grow indoors when sufficient moisture is available. Exposure to microbial contaminants is clinically associated with respiratory symptoms, allergies, asthma and immunological reactions.

Indoor air plays a special role as a health determinant, and management of indoor air quality requires approaches that differ from those used for outdoor air. For these reasons, the working group preparing the global update of the WHO air quality guidelines (WHO Regional Office for Europe, 2006a) recommended that WHO also prepare guidelines for indoor air quality. This is in line with the recommendations of an earlier WHO working group that formulated *The right to healthy indoor air* and, in particular, with its Principle 6, which states that "Under the principle of accountability, all relevant organizations should establish explicit criteria for evaluating and assessing building air quality and its impact on the health of the population and on the environment" (WHO Regional Office for Europe, 2000a).

The subsequent working group meeting in Bonn in October 2006 acknowledged the applicability of the existing WHO guidelines for air quality (WHO Regional Office for Europe, 2000b, 2006a) to indoor air and identified a number of chemical substances for which specific indoor air guidelines was recommended. The working group also recommended guidelines for two additional categories of risk factors of particular importance to health in indoor environments: biological agents and indoor combustion (WHO Regional Office for Europe, 2006b).

Biological agents of relevance to health are widely heterogeneous, ranging from pollen and spores of plants (mainly from outdoors), to bacteria, fungi, algae and some protozoa emitted outdoors or indoors. They also include a wide variety of microbes and allergens that spread from person to person. There is strong evidence regarding the hazards posed by several biological agents that pollute indoor air; however, the WHO working group convened in October 2006 concluded that the individual species of microbes and other biological agents that are responsible for health effects cannot be identified. This is due to people often being exposed to multiple agents simultaneously, to complexities in accurate estimation of exposure and to the large numbers of symptoms and health outcomes due to exposure. The exceptions include some common allergies, which can be attributed to specific agents, such as house dust mites and pets.

While quantitative guidelines could not be provided for the concentrations of many biological agents, recommendations, guidance or guidelines (all referred to 'guidelines' in this text) have been formulated to protect health and identify health risks by defining indicators of a safe indoor environment. Thus, the guidelines define problems and the circumstances in which risk is likely to occur but do not include recommendations on acceptable levels of exposure to biological agents. The aim of these guidelines is to help public health authorities and the general public to identify the hazards and reduce the risks. They do not, however,

---

BOX 1   Definitions of some terms used in the guidelines

Air-conditioning system: assembly of equipment for treating air to control simultaneously its temperature, humidity, cleanliness and distribution to meet the requirements of a conditioned space.

Dampness: any visible, measurable or perceived outcome of excess moisture that causes problems in buildings, such as mould, leaks or material degradation, mould odour or directly measured excess moisture (in terms of relative humidity or moisture content) or microbial growth.

Excess moisture: moisture state variable that is higher than a design criterion, usually represented as moisture content or relative humidity in building material or the air. Design criteria can be simple indicators (e.g. no condensation or relative humidity value) or more complicated representations that take into account continuous fluctuation of moisture (i.e. mould growth index).

Moisture: (1) water vapour; (2) water in a medium, such as soil or insulation, but not bulk water or flowing water.

Moisture problem or damage; water damage: any visible, measurable or perceived outcome caused by excess moisture indicating indoor climate problems or problems of durability in building assemblies; moisture damage is a particular problem of building assembly durability; water damage is a moisture problem caused by various leaks of water.

Moisture transport: moisture can be transported in both the vapour and the liquid phase by diffusion, convection, capillary suction, wind pressure and gravity (water pressure).

Mould: all species of microscopic fungi that grow in the form of multicellular filaments, called hyphae. In contrast, microscopic fungi that grow as single cells are called *yeasts*, a connected network of tubular branching hyphae has multiple, genetically identical nuclei and is considered a single organism, referred to as a *colony* (Madigan, Martinko, 2005).

Ventilation: process of supplying or removing air by natural or mechanical means to or from any space; the air may or may not have been conditioned.

make recommendations for specific actions to manage indoor air quality, which must be addressed at the national or local level, as has already been done in some countries.

Although the literature on biological contaminants in indoor air is vast, there is no universal agreement on the precise meaning of the terms used to describe the (micro-)environmental conditions determining their presence and proliferation. The definitions used in these guidelines are shown in Box 1.

The presence of many biological agents in indoor environments is attributable to dampness and inadequate ventilation. Excess moisture on almost all indoor materials leads to growth of microbes, such as mould, fungi and bacteria, which subsequently emit spores, cells, fragments and volatile organic compounds into indoor air. Moreover, dampness initiates chemical or biological degradation of materials, which also pollute indoor air. Dampness has therefore been suggested to be strong, consistent indicator of risk of asthma and respiratory symptoms (e.g. cough and wheeze). The health risks of biological contaminants of indoor air could thus be addressed by considering dampness as the risk indicator.

Several widely acknowledged global trends contribute to the conditions associated with increased exposure to dampness and mould:

- energy conservation measures that are not properly implemented (tightened building envelopes, ventilation deficits, improper insulation);
- urbanization (migration, building type and density, urban degradation, housing availability and social inequity);
- climate change (increasing frequency of extreme weather conditions, shifting of climate zones); and
- the quality and globalization of building materials and components, construction concepts and techniques.

These conditions increase the risks of adverse health effects due to biological contaminants of indoor air.

1.2   Scope of the review

One of the recommendations of the WHO working group that met in October 2006 was to identify the main health risks due to dampness, the associated microbial growth and contamination of indoor spaces and to formulate relevant guidelines for the protection of public health. As separate guidelines are to be prepared specifically for allergens from pets and from house-dust mites, these aspects are mentioned only briefly in these guidelines and only if moisture and dampness determine their presence.

The review covers not only mould but also covers to some extent other biological agents, such as bacteria associated with excess moisture in indoor environments. As it was not feasible to include all the exposure factors in the title,

Figure 1. Pathways linking sources of dampness with health

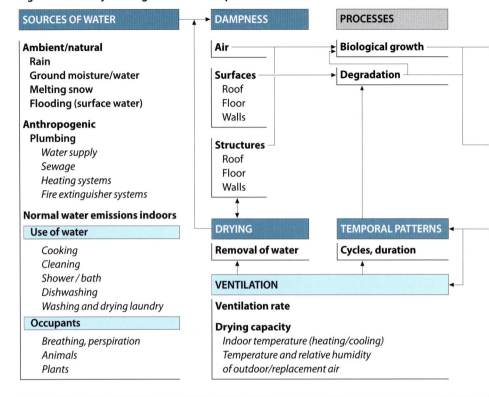

dampness and mould were accepted as a compromise between brevity and precision concerning the content of the guidelines.

The need for definitions of terms such as *dampness* and *moisture* was discussed extensively during the review. The working group agreed, however, that while it is important to use terms consistently, explicit definitions have limitations. In the scientific studies reviewed, various definitions were used, and even native language speakers could not recognize subtle differences in the different definitions. Therefore, the terms used had to be evaluated separately in each context.

The complex causal chain of events that constitute a health hazard links sources of water through excessive moisture to biological growth and physical and chemical degradation and further to emission of hazardous biological and chemical agents (Figure 1). The review of evidence follows this chain, summarizing the issues related to building dampness and its impacts on indoor exposure to biological and non-biological pollutants in Chapter 2, which also presents approaches to exposure assessment.

An important determinant of dampness and biological growth in indoor spaces is ventilation, which is discussed in Chapter 3. The working group acknowledged that ventilation plays a major role in building operation and occu-

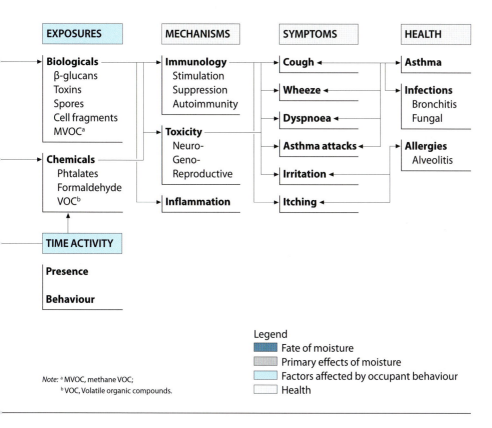

| EXPOSURES | MECHANISMS | SYMPTOMS | HEALTH |

Biologicals
β-glucans
Toxins
Spores
Cell fragments
MVOC[a]

Chemicals
Phtalates
Formaldehyde
VOC[b]

TIME ACTIVITY

Presence

Behaviour

Immunology
Stimulation
Suppression
Autoimmunity

Toxicity
Neuro-
Geno-
Reproductive

Inflammation

Cough

Wheeze

Dyspnoea

Asthma attacks

Irritation

Itching

Asthma

Infections
Bronchitis
Fungal

Allergies
Alveolitis

Legend
Fate of moisture
Primary effects of moisture
Factors affected by occupant behaviour
Health

Note: [a] MVOC, methane VOC;
     [b] VOC, Volatile organic compounds.

pants' health and that these aspects should be covered in another volume of the *Indoor air quality guidelines* (e.g. in guidelines on indoor combustion). Moisture control in building structures is the second important issue summarized in Chapter 3. Unfavourable combinations of air humidity and temperature differences in building structures may lead to condensation of water on surfaces and consequent decomposition of building materials and microbial growth.

The evidence for the health effects of indoor exposure to dampness and mould is presented in Chapter 4, which is based on reviews of epidemiological studies and clinical and toxicological research.

1.3   Preparation of the guidelines

The planning meeting in 2006 recommended that a steering group[2] be established to guide preparation of the guidelines. The group recommended potential authors and reviewers for the first draft of the background material, which was submitted to WHO in August 2007 and, after compilation, distributed for

---

[2] Steering group members: Ross Anderson, Aaron Cohen, Séverine Kirchner, Lars Mølhave, Aino Nevalainen, Bernd Seifert, Kirk Smith and John Spengler

external review. The drafts and the reviewers' comments provided the background for the discussions of the WHO working group meeting in Bonn, 17–18 October 2007, which evaluated both the scientific evidence and the comments made in the review. The working group then summarized their evaluations of the health risks and recommended the guidelines presented in Chapter 5 of this document. The comments collected before and during the working group meeting were used by the primary authors of the background material to prepare the second drafts of Chapters 1–4. These drafts were reviewed by the working group members. The final versions of the chapters incorporated the comments of all reviewers and were accepted by the steering group.

It is anticipated that the recommendations in these guidelines will remain valid until 2018. The Department of Public Health and Environment at WHO headquarters in Geneva will be responsible for initiating a review of these guidelines at that time.

1.4   Guidelines and indoor air quality management

The guidelines are intended for worldwide use, to protect public health under various environmental, social and economic conditions and to support the achievement of optimal indoor air quality. They focus on building characteristics that prevent the occurrence of adverse health effects associated with dampness or mould. The guidelines are applicable to various levels of economic development and different climates, cover all relevant population groups, and propose feasible approaches to reducing health risks due to dampness and microbial contamination. Chapters 2–4 summarize the scientific evidence on the relationships between dampness, mould and health effects. Both private and public buildings (e.g. offices and nursing homes) are covered, as dampness and mould are risks everywhere. Settings with particular production processes and hospitals with high-risk patients or sources of exposure to pathogens are not, however, considered.

While the guidelines provide objectives for indoor air quality management, they do not give instructions for achieving those objectives. The necessary action and indicators depend on local technical conditions, the level of development, human capacities and resources. The guidelines recommended by WHO acknowledge this heterogeneity. In formulating policy targets, governments should consider their local circumstances and select actions that will ensure achievement of their health objectives most effectively.

2. Building dampness and its effect on indoor exposure to biological and non-biological pollutants

Jeroen Douwes

2.1 Frequency of indoor dampness

A review of studies in several European countries, Canada and the United States in 2004 indicated that at least 20% of buildings had one or more signs of dampness (Institute of Medicine, 2004). This estimate agrees with those of a study of 16 190 people in Denmark, Estonia, Iceland, Norway and Sweden, which gave an overall prevalence of indoor dampness of 18%, with the lowest prevalence in Göteborg, Sweden (12.1%), and the highest in Tartu, Estonia (31.6%) (Gunnbjörnsdóttir et al., 2006). Dampness was defined on the basis of self-reported indicators, such as water leakage or damage, bubbles or discoloration of floor coverings, and visible mould growth indoors on walls, floors or ceilings. From several studies conducted in the United States, Mudarri and Fisk (2007) estimated the prevalence of dampness or mould in houses to be approximately 50%.

Although few data are available for low-income countries, several studies suggest that indoor dampness is also common in other areas of the world. For example, a study of 4164 children in rural Taiwan, China, showed that 12.2% of the parents or guardians considered their dwelling to be damp, 30.1% reported the presence of visible mould inside the house in the past year, 43.4% reported the appearance of standing water, water damage or leaks, and 60% reported at least one of these occurrences (Yang et al., 1997a). In a study in Singapore of 4759 children, the prevalence of dampness in the child's bedroom was 5% and that of mould was 3% (Tham et al., 2007); the overall prevalence of mould and damp in the rest of the house was not given. About 11% of parents of 10 902 schoolchildren in a study in three cities in China (Beijing, Guangzhou and Hong Kong Special Administrative Region) reported mould on the ceilings and walls (Wong et al., 2004). In a study in Japan of the residents of 98 houses built within the past 4 years, condensation on window panes or walls was reported by the residents in 41.7% of all houses, and 15.6% had visible mould (Saijo et al., 2004). Indoor damp was reported by 13% of 3368 adults living in Nikel in the Arctic area of the northern Russian Federation (Dotterud, Falk, 1999). A case-control study of asthma in the West Bank and Gaza Strip, involving participants in villages, cities and refugee camps, showed that 62 of 110 dwellings (56%) had visible mould on the walls and ceilings (El Sharif et al., 2004). The prevalence of houses characterized as damp with visible mould was highest in the refugee camps, with an estimated 75% of houses affected. Another study in the West Bank in 188 randomly selected houses in the Al-Ama'ri refugee camp south of Ramallah City showed that 78.2% of the houses had damp problems, leaks or indoor mould (Al-Khatib et al., 2003).

As dampness is more likely to occur in houses that are overcrowded and lack appropriate heating, ventilation and insulation (Institute of Medicine 2004), the prevalence of indoor damp in low-income communities can be substantially higher than the national average. For example, in a study of 1954 young mothers in the United Kingdom, those who lived in owner-occupied or mortgaged accommodations (relatively affluent) reported damp (52%) and mould (24%) significantly less often than those who lived in council houses or rented accommodations (relatively deprived), 58% of whom reported damp and 56% of whom reported mould (Baker, Henderson, 1999). Similarly, a study of 25 864 schoolchildren in eastern Germany showed that the children of parents with a low educational level were 4.8 times more likely (95% confidence interval (CI), 3.4–5.4) to live in damp houses than those of parents with a high level of education. Children whose parents had received education at the intermediate level were 1.8 times as likely to live in a damp house (95% CI, 1.6–2.1) (du Prel, Kramer, Ranft, 2005).

Indoor damp is likely to remain an important issue in less affluent countries and neighbourhoods, particularly since an increasing shortage of affordable housing provides little incentive for landlords to improve rental accommodation. Similarly, the substantial costs involved in remediation may dissuade low-income home owners from improving substandard housing conditions. This will add to the already high burden of poor health in those communities.

Most of the estimates of prevalence are based on self-reports and may therefore be biased. To address this problem, self-reports of dampness were compared in several studies with results obtained through inspections by trained personnel. Although in most of these studies the occupants reported more dampness than the trained surveyors (Bornehag et al., 2001), some studies showed that occupants reported less dampness (Williamson et al., 1997; Nevalainen et al., 1998). Studies by Engman, Bornehag and Sundell (2007) and Sun, Sundhell and Zhang (2007) also showed poor agreement between self-reported and inspectors' observations of dampness and mouldy odour. Douwes et al. (1999), however, found that occupants' reports of damp spots or fungal spots correlated better with an objective measure of indoor fungi than investigators' reports of these visible signs; a similar finding was reported by Sun, Sundhell and Zhang (2007). This result was not confirmed by another study, in which objective measures of fungal concentrations and questionnaire reports were compared (Dales, Miller, McMullen, 1997).

The exact prevalence of home dampness cannot be established in the absence of a gold standard, but occupants' and inspectors' reports indicate that it is likely to be in the order of 10–50% in the most affluent countries. Although the evidence is more limited for less affluent countries, the magnitude of the problem appears to be similar, the prevalence sometimes even exceeding 50% (e.g. in refugee camps in the West Bank and Gaza Strip, see above). As problems of damp are commonest in deprived neighbourhoods, a substantial proportion of that population is at risk of adverse health effects associated with damp indoor environments (see Chapter 4).

Climate change and its effects on the weather (i.e. storms and heavy rainfall) and the subsequent rise in sea level and increased frequency and duration of floods are likely to increase the proportion of buildings with damp problems further, particularly in flood-prone areas such as river valleys and coastal areas. In addition, high energy costs will prevent adequate heating in winter in many houses (so-called fuel poverty), leading to increased condensation and indoor dampness.

Dampness and indoor mould also occur in school buildings, day-care centres, offices and other buildings (Mudarri, Fisk, 2007). The health risks associated with dampness-related exposures in these building are likely to be similar to those in damp houses; however, no systematic surveys have been conducted to assess the prevalence of dampness and mould in these establishments.

2.2 Effects of dampness on the quality of the indoor environment

Indoor environments contain a complex mixture of live (viable) and dead (non-viable) microorganisms, fragments thereof, toxins, allergens, volatile microbial organic compounds and other chemicals. The indoor concentrations of some of these organisms and agents are known or suspected to be elevated in damp indoor environments and may affect the health of people living or working there (see Chapter 4). In particular, it has been suggested that dust mites and fungi, both of which favour damp environments, play a major role. Dust mites and several fungi produce allergens known to be associated with allergies and asthma; many fungi also produce toxins and irritants with suspected effects on respiratory health.

Dampness may also promote bacterial growth and the survival of viruses, but this has received little attention in the literature (see sections 2.3.2 and 2.3.7). In addition, dampness is an indicator of poor ventilation, which may result in increased levels of a wide range of other potentially harmful indoor pollutants (see Chapter 3). Excess moisture may also result in increased chemical emissions from building materials and floor covers (see section 2.3.6). Furthermore, standing water may attract cockroaches and rodents, which can transmit infectious diseases and are also a source of indoor allergens. These pests are not specific to damp buildings, however, and are therefore not be discussed further in this document. Damp indoor environments (particularly damp soil and wood) may also attract termites, which can cause substantial damage to buildings, significantly compromising the integrity of the structure and therefore the health and safety of its occupants. Also, the presence of termites may indirectly affect the indoor environment by inducing the use (and misuse) of potentially hazardous pesticides. As termites are not known to affect indoor air quality directly, they are not discussed further in this document. Although outbreaks of legionellosis are commonly associated with water sources in buildings, they are not typically associated with damp buildings and are also not discussed further.

2.2.1 Dust mites

As indicated in Chapter 1, the focus of these guidelines is dampness, mould and microbial agents (see below). The close association between damp indoor environments and dust mites is, however, discussed briefly. The reader is referred to the report of the Institute of Medicine (2000) on house dampness and asthma for a more detailed overview of the literature on the associations between indoor damp, house dust mite allergens and asthma.

House dust mites are arachnids, and many different species have been identified; however, only a few are of concern with respect to damp indoor environments (see section 2.3.1). The natural food source of house-dust mites includes skin scales, although many other sources may be used. Therefore, in most houses, nutrition is abundantly available, particularly in mattresses and carpets or rugs. Laboratory studies have shown that most dust mites require a relative humidity in excess of 45–50% for survival and development, but they feed and multiply more rapidly at higher relative humidity (Arlian, 1992). Indoor humidity is therefore the main influence on the presence and propagation of house dust mites, as confirmed in several field studies (van Strien et al., 1994; de Andrade et al., 1995; Simpson et al., 2002; van Strien et al., 2004; Zock et al., 2006). Damp houses therefore significantly increase exposure to dust-mite allergens, at least in populations living in mild and temperate climates.

2.2.2 Fungi

Fungi are ubiquitous eukaryotic organisms, comprising an abundance of species. They may be transported into buildings on the surface of new materials or on clothing. They may also penetrate buildings through active or passive ventilation. Fungi are therefore found in the dust and surfaces of every house, including those with no problems with damp. Once fungi are indoors, fungal growth can occur only in the presence of moisture, and many fungi grow readily on any surface that becomes wet or moistened; that is, virtually all fungi readily germinate and grow on substrates in equilibrium with a relative humidity below saturation (i.e. below 100%).

The species that grow on a given substrate depends largely on the water activity of the substrate. Water activity is a measure of water availability and is defined as the ratio of the vapour pressure above a substrate relative to that above pure water measured at the same temperature and pressure. The minimum water activity required for fungal growth on building surfaces varies from less than 0.80 to greater than 0.98 (Grant et al., 1989; see also Table 1). On the basis of their water requirements, indoor fungi can be divided into: (1) primary colonizers, which can grow at a water activity less than or equal to 0.80; (2) secondary colonizers, which grow at a water activity level of 0.80–0.90; and (3) tertiary colonizers, which require a water activity greater than 0.90 to germinate and start mycelial growth (Grant et al., 1989; see also Table 1). Although high levels of humidity and some surface and interstitial condensation may be sufficient for most primary and secondary colonizers, tertiary colonizers generally require serious condensation problems. These problems may be due to construction faults, including inadequate insulation, in combination with poor ventilation, or water damage from leaks, flooding and groundwater intrusion.

Fungi also need nutrients, which may include carbohydrates, proteins and lipids. The sources are diverse and plentiful, ranging from plant or animal matter in house dust to surface and construction materials (such as wallpaper and textiles), condensation or deposition of cooking oils, paint and glue, wood, stored products (such as food), and books and other paper products. Nutrients are therefore generally not a limiting factor for indoor fungal growth. In fact, fungi are known to grow even on inert materials such as ceramic tiles and can obtain sufficient nutrients from dust particles and soluble components of water. As most indoor fungi grow at 10–35 °C, common indoor temperatures are also not a limiting factor; however, although temperature and nutrients are not critical, they may affect the rate of growth (see section 3.3) and the production of certain allergens and metabolites (Nielsen et al., 1999; Institute of Medicine, 2000). Thus, water remains the most critical factor in indoor fungal growth, as also indicated in field studies, which show elevated numbers of fungi and fungal spores in damp houses (Gallup et al., 1987; Waegemaekers et al., 1989; Douwes et al., 1999). House dampness therefore significantly contributes to fungal spores, fragments and allergens (see section 2.3).

Fungi not only have adverse effects on health but also cause considerable damage to buildings, the wood-rotting fungi being particularly destructive to (wooden) building structures. The commonest and possibly the most destructive wood decay fungus found in buildings in temperate regions, including Australia, Europe and Japan, is the dry-rot fungus *Serpula lacrymans* (previously known as *Merulius lacrymans*) (Singh, 1999). This fungus can grow quickly and may spread throughout a building from one timber to another, potentially causing devastating effects in the whole building. There are many other dry- and wet-rot fungi that can cause wood decay and subsequent damage to the built environment (reviewed by Singh, 1999). They have also been implicated in the causation of hypersensitivity pneumonitis (extrinsic allergic alveolitis).

Table 1. Moisture levels required for growth of selected microorganisms in construction, finishing and furnishing materials

Moisture level	Category of microorganism
High (a$_w$, > 0.90; ERH, > 90%)	Tertiary colonizers (hydrophilic) *Alternaria alternata* *Aspergillus fumigatus* *Epicoccum* spp. *Exophiala* spp. *Fusarium moniliforme* *Mucor plumbeus* *Phoma herbarum* *Phialophora* spp. *Rhizopus* spp. *Stachybotrys chartarum* (*S. atra*) *Trichoderma* spp. *Ulocladium consortiale* *Rhodotorula* spp. *Sporobolomyces* spp. Actinobacteria (or Actinomycetes)
Intermediate (a$_w$, 0.80–0.90; ERH, 80–90%)	Secondary colonizers *Aspergillus flavus* *Aspergillus versicolor*[a] *Cladosporium cladosporioides* *Cladosporium herbarum* *Cladosporium sphaerospermum* *Mucor circinelloides* *Rhizopus oryzae*
Low (a$_w$, < 0.80; ERH, < 80%)	Primary colonizers (xerophilic) *Alternaria citri* *Aspergillus (Eurotium) amstelodami* *Aspergillus candidus* *Aspergillus (Eurotium) glaucus* *Aspergillus niger* *Aspergillus penicillioides* *Aspergillus (Eurotium) repens* *Aspergillus restrictus* *Aspergillus versicolor*[b] *Paecilomyces variotii* *Penicillium aurantiogriseum* *Penicillium brevicompactum* *Penicillium chrysogenum* *Penicillium commune* *Penicillium expansum* *Penicillium griseofulvum* *Wallemia sebi*

Note. a$_w$, water activity; ERH, equilibrium relative humidity
Sources: Grant et al. (1989); Gravesen, Frisvad, Samson (1994); ISIAQ (1996)
[a] at 12 °C; [b] at 25 °C

2.2.3 Bacteria

Bacteria are ubiquitous prokaryotic single-cell organisms, comprising an abundance of species. They can be found in the dust and on the surfaces of every house, including those with no damp problems. The main sources of bacteria in the indoor environment are outdoor air, people and indoor bacterial growth. Bacteria from outdoor air and those originating from people are considered to be fairly harmless; bacteria growing actively or accumulating in the indoor environment, however, may affect health, but this has not been studied extensively.

As described for fungi, water is a critical requirement for bacterial growth. In fact, bacteria require higher water activities than most fungi. The temperature and nutrient demands are generally met in most indoor environments. Surprisingly, few studies have been conducted on bacterial growth in damp houses. Those that have suggest that bacteria grow in the same areas as fungi. In particular, *Streptomycetes* (Gram-positive spore-forming bacteria that are not normal indoor flora in urban environments) may grow on damp or wet building materials (Hyvärinen et al., 2002). Their presence in indoor air may therefore indicate that a building has a moisture problem (Samson et al., 1994). Although no clear association with dampness has been found, it has been suggested that endotoxins from Gram-negative bacteria occur at increased levels in damp buildings (Bischof et al., 2002; Solomon et al., 2006).

2.2.4 Protozoa

It has been proposed that protozoa play a role in the complex mixture of exposures that contribute to adverse health effects associated with damp indoor environments (Yli-Pirila et al., 2004). In their study, amoeba were detected in 22% of 124 material samples from moisture-damaged buildings. Most of the 11 samples of materials that were badly damaged by moisture were found to contain ciliates and flagellates. No field studies have been conducted to assess the airborne concentrations of protozoa or fragments thereof. Although a study in vitro suggested that amoeba enhance the pro-inflammatory properties of certain microbes (Yli-Pirila et al., 2007), it is not clear whether protozoa in damp buildings contribute to ill health.

2.3 Dampness-related indoor pollutants

In this section, we describe the most important indoor pollutants that have been associated with damp indoor spaces and related health effects. The health effects associated with these pollutants are discussed in Chapter 4.

2.3.1 Allergens

All agents that can induce specific immune responses (resulting in the production of specific antibodies) are also potential allergens. The term *allergen* can refer to a single molecule, a mixture of molecules or a particle from which allergen molecules can be eluted. The latter can be dead material, like mite faecal particles, or viable propagules, such as bacteria or mould spores. Thus, allergens comprise a large variety of macromolecular structures, ranging from low-relative-molecular-mass sensitizers (mainly chemicals such as formaldehyde) to high-relativemolecular- mass sensitizers (such as polymeric carbohydrates and proteins). In damp indoor environments, those with a high relative molecular mass are most relevant, in particular house dust mite allergens and fungal allergens.

2.3.1.1. House dust mite allergens

Dust mites produce the predominant inhalation allergens in many parts of the world. The most common mite species that produce allergens are *Dermatophagoides pteronyssinus* and *Dermatophagoides farinae*. The major allergens produced by *D. pteronyssisus* (called Der p I and Der p II) are proteases, which are present in large amounts in faecal pellets (Institute of Medicine, 2000). The major allergen produced by *D. farinae* is Der f I. Elevated levels of these allergens have been detected in house dust, mattress dust and bedding in damp houses (van Strien et al., 1994; Simpson et al., 2002; van Strien et al., 2004). As the focus of these guidelines is indoor dampness and microorganisms, dust mite allergen levels are not discussed further.

2.3.1.2. Fungal allergens

Many fungal species produce type I allergens, and immunoglobulin (Ig)E sensitization to the commonest outdoor and indoor fungal species, like *Alternaria*, *Penicillium*, *Aspergillus* and *Cladosporium* spp., is strongly associated with allergic respiratory disease, especially asthma (Chapter 4). Fungi are also well-known sources of type III (or IgG-inducing) allergens. The species involved include many common genera such as *Penicillium* and *Aspergillus*, which can be found in most houses. At high concentrations, fungi may also be involved in combined type III and IV allergic reactions, including hypersensitivity pneumonitis.

Many fungal allergens are glycopeptides with enzymatic properties. They are found in spores, hyphae and fungal fragments but are released in greater amounts during germination and mycelial growth, which may occur inside the airways (Green et al., 2006). The viability of spores is therefore important for allergenic expression, as confirmed in some studies in experimental animals. Although non-viable fungal spores and hyphae release allergens at lower concentrations, they are still likely to play an important role in fungi-related allergies and respiratory effects. Non-viable fungal spores and fungal fragments also contain potentially harmful compounds such as $(1\rightarrow3)$-β-D-glucans and mycotoxins (see sections 2.3.4 and 2.3.5). Species of the genera *Cladosporium*, *Alternaria* and *Aspergillus* have been shown to produce a variety of allergens, including several major ones: Cla h I (*Cladosporum herbarum*), Alt a I and Alt a II (*Alternaria alternata*) and Asp f I and Asp f III (*Aspergillus fumigatus*). Nonetheless, the most potent allergenic proteins, identified as *major allergens* in fungal extracts produced in vitro, might not be the same as those to which people are actually exposed in indoor environments. This might explain the negative skin-prick test and IgE results in people with asthma (see Chapter 4).

Commercial assays are available for only a limited number of indoor fungal allergens (including *Alternaria* allergens, see section 2.4.3) because of difficulties in the manufacture and standardization of fungal allergen extracts. Therefore, little information is available on exposure to these allergens.

Many fungi and some yeast replicate by producing numerous spores that are well adapted to airborne dispersal. Spores are typically 2–10 µm in length. They can stay airborne for long periods and may deposit in the respiratory system, some smaller spores reaching the alveoli (Eduard, 2006). Fungi also release even smaller fungal fragments (Gorny, 2004), which are derived from broken or fractured spores and hyphae and can be categorized into submicron particles (< 1 µm) or larger fungal fragments (> 1 µm). Even more fungal fragments than spores may be deposited in the respiratory tract (Cho et al., 2005); like spores, they are known to contain allergens (Green et al., 2006) and mycotoxins (Brasel et al., 2005a). Both spores and fungal fragments may therefore be involved in mould-related adverse health effects.

The aerosolization of fungal matter and its subsequent inhalation are only partly understood, but two mechanisms are believed to be of particular importance: (1) release of spores or fungal fragments by active discharge, indoor air movement or physical disturbance caused by people or pets; and (2) resuspension of settled fungal matter due to human activities. Factors that may affect the rate of release of spores or fungal fragments include air velocity, time, colony structure, desiccation stress, moisture condition and vibration. These factors may affect the rate of aerosolization of spores and fungal fragments differently (Gorny, 2004).

Fungal spores are ubiquitous in outdoor air, the levels ranging from less than 100 to more than 10^5 spores/m^3. The indoor levels are usually lower than those outdoors but may be increased by unintended fungal growth in damp buildings (Flannigan, Samson, Miller, 2001). Studies in damp indoor environments have shown a wide diversity of fungal species and genera, probably due to differences in climate, indoor temperature and humidity, and building materials, as well as differences in sample collection and subsequent culture. Fungi are often found on wet window frames and damp walls of bedrooms, living rooms and kitchens. Mattresses constitute an important reservoir for mould, with measured concentrations of 10^3–10^7 spores/g of dust (Verhoeff et al., 1994a). Several extensive reviews on fungal species found in damp indoor environments have been published (e.g. Flannigan, Samson, Miller, 2001).

The airborne concentrations of viable fungi in indoor environments are usually in the order of a few to several thousand colony-forming units (CFUs) per cubic metre of air. In a given space, concentrations of fungi are highly variable and depend on such factors as: climate and season, type of fungus, construction, age and use of the building, and ventilation rate. They also depend largely on the sampling and analytical methods used, making valid comparisons between studies difficult.

Indoor fungal fragments are not commonly measured in field studies, but a study with an aerosolization chamber showed that submicron fungal fragments from culture plates and mould-contaminated ceiling tiles aerosolized simultaneously with spores but at substantially higher concentrations (320–514 times higher) (Gorny et al., 2002; Cho et al., 2005). This suggests that indoor exposure to fungal fragments is at least as important as exposure to fungal spores.

2.3.2 Bacteria

As mentioned above, few studies have addressed bacteria in damp indoor environments. Some identified *Streptomycetes* on damp or wet indoor surfaces (Hyvärinen et al., 2002; Rintala, Nevalainen, Suutari, 2002; Rintala et al., 2004). *Streptomycetes* are Gram-positive, spore-forming actinobacteria, which are typical soil organisms that produce a wide range of metabolites, including some toxins, such as valinomycin (Andersson et al., 1998). The metabolites produced are substrate-dependent (Hirvonen et al., 2001; Roponen et al., 2001; Murtoniemi et al., 2001a, 2003). Mycobacteria have also been shown to be common in moisture damaged buildings, their presence increasing with the degree of fungal damage (Torvinen et al., 2006). Cell wall components of mycobacteria are known to be highly immunogenic, and exposure to mycobacteria may cause inflammatory responses (Huttunen et al., 2000, 2001).

The concentrations of total viable bacteria in indoor environments may range between 10^1 and 10^3 CFU/m^3 (Gorny, Dutkiewicz, Krysinska-Traczyk, 1999), probably representing the degree of occupancy of the building and the efficiency of its ventilation. The literature does not provide typical airborne concentrations in damp indoor environments as compared with non-damp environments. Also, although the presence of *Streptomycetes* and mycobacteria may be an indication of bacterial growth, normal levels have not been established.

2.3.3 Endotoxins

Endotoxins are integral components of the outer membrane of Gram-negative bacteria and are composed of proteins, lipids and lipopolysaccharides. The term *endotoxin* refers to a toxin on the bacterial cell wall, which is often liberated as a result of cell lysis. In the environment, airborne endotoxins are usually associated with dust particles or aqueous aerosols. They have a broad size distribution, but the levels may be higher in the coarse fraction (Schwarze et al., 2007). Heavy exposure to endotoxins can cause respiratory symptoms, including non-allergic asthma, but moderate-to-low exposure may protect against allergies and asthma

(Douwes, Pearce, Heederik, 2002). It has been hypothesized that endotoxins play a role in the pathogenisis of rheumatic diseases in damp buildings (Lorenz et al., 2006).

Lipopolysaccharides are a class of pure lipid carbohydrate molecules (free of protein and other cell-wall components) and are responsible for most of the immunological properties of bacterial endotoxins. Lipopolysaccharides are stable, water-soluble, non-allergenic molecules composed of a lipid and a polysaccharide and have not been found in the cell walls of Gram-positive bacteria, mycobacteria or fungi (Morrison, Ryan, 1979; Rietschel et al., 1985). The lipid moiety of lipopolysaccharides, called *lipid A*, is responsible for their toxic properties. Although the terms *endotoxins* and *lipopolysaccharides* technically have different meanings, they are often used interchangeably in the scientific literature.

The concentrations of endotoxins in the indoor environment range from a few to several thousand endotoxin units per milligram of house dust (Douwes, Pearce, Heederik, 2002). When the concentration is expressed per square metre, it varies even more. The endotoxin levels in different studies vary only moderately, regardless of the geographical area, which is remarkable, as the analytical methods used were not standardized. Few studies have focused on airborne concentrations in the indoor environment. Park et al. (2000) reported a mean airborne endotoxin level of 0.64 units/m^3 in 15 houses in Boston, United States, and mean levels of endotoxins in dust of 44–105 units/mg. The mean inhalable level of endotoxins measured in nine houses in Belgium was similar, i.e. 0.24 units/m^3 (Bouillard, Devleeschouwer, Michel, 2006). Indoor concentrations may be higher in damp houses, but a study conducted in areas of Louisiana affected by hurricane Katrina and the subsequent flooding did not confirm this (Solomon et al., 2006). Other studies also found no evidence for a relationship between endotoxins in house dust and observed dampness or mould (Chen et al., 2007; Giovannangelo et al., 2007).

2.3.4 Fungal (1→3)-β-D-glucans

(1→3)-β-D-glucans are non-allergenic, water-insoluble structural cell-wall components of most fungi, some bacteria, most higher plants and many lower plants (Stone, Clarke, 1992). They consist of glucose polymers with variable relative molecular mass and degree of branching (Williams, 1997) and may account for up to 60% of the dry weight of the cell wall of fungi (Klis, 1994). In the fungal cell wall, (1→3)-β-D-glucans are linked to proteins, lipids and carbohydrates such as mannan and chitin, and they contain (1→6)-β-glucan side-branches, which may connect with adjacent (1→3)-β-D-glucan polymers (Klis, 1994). The (1→3)-β-D-glucan content of fungal cell walls has been reported to be relatively independent of growth conditions (Rylander, 1997a; Foto et al., 2004). (1→3)-β-D-glucans have immunomodulating properties and may affect respiratory health (Douwes, 2005; see also section 4.2.1).

The methods used to analyse $(1\rightarrow3)$-β-D-glucans in environmental (settled or airborne) dust samples have not been standardized, and studies are therefore not comparable. In Sweden and Switzerland, the concentrations in buildings with fungal problems ranged from about 10 to more than 100 ng/m³ in a *Limulus* amoebocyte lysate assay in airborne dust samples generated by rigorous agitation of settled dust in the buildings (Rylander, 1999) (see section 2.4 for a description of analytical methods). The concentrations in buildings with no obvious fungal problems were close to 1 ng/m³. The mean levels of $(1\rightarrow3)$-β-D-glucans in house dust in Germany and the Netherlands, determined with a specific enzyme immunoassay, were comparable: 1000–2000 µg/g dust and 500–1000 µg/m² (Douwes et al., 1996, 1998, 2000; Gehring et al., 2001; Chew et al., 2001). Samples were taken in houses that were not selected because of fungal problems and were analysed in the same laboratory with identical procedures. No airborne samples were taken.

2.3.5   Mycotoxins

Mycotoxins, or fungal toxins, are low-relative-molecular-mass biomolecules produced by fungi, some of which are toxic to animals and human beings. Mycotoxins are known to interfere with RNA synthesis and may cause DNA damage. Some fungal species may produce various mycotoxins, depending on the substrate. In the case of *Penicillium*, one such compound is penicillin, a strong antibiotic. Several mycotoxins, e.g. aflatoxin from *Aspergillus flavus* and *Aspergillus parasiticus*, are potent carcinogens. Many mycotoxins are immunotoxic, but the trichothecene mycotoxins are immunostimulating at low doses (Eduard, 2006). Numerous mycotoxins have been classified by their distinct chemical structures and reactive functional groups, including primary and secondary amines, hydroxyl or phenolic groups, lactams, carboxylic acids, and amides.

The mycotoxins that have perhaps received most attention are the trichothecenes, produced by *Stachybotrys chartarum*. Bloom et al. (2007) showed that several mycotoxins produced by *S. chartarum* and *Aspergillus versicolor* (i.e. macrocyclic trichothecenes, trichodermin, sterigmatocystin and satratoxin G) could be present in most samples of materials and settled dust from buildings with current or past damage from damp or water. Charpin-Kadouch et al. (2006) compared the levels of macrocyclic trichothecenes in samples from 15 flooded dwellings known to be contaminated with *S. chartarum* or *Chaetomium,* and a group of nine dwellings without visible mould. The level of macrocyclic trichothecenes was significantly higher in floor dust from the mouldy houses than from the reference dwellings; the levels in wall samples from mouldy houses were also higher (of borderline statistical significance), but no statistically significant difference in air concentrations was observed. In a study by Brasel et al. (2005a) in seven buildings known to be contaminated with *S. chartarum*, the airborne level of macrocyclic trichothecenes was significantly higher than that in four control buildings (i.e. with no detectable *S. chartarum* or history of water damage). The same authors also showed that *S. chartarum* trichothecene mycotoxins can become airborne in association with both intact conidia and smaller fungal fragments (Brasel et al., 2005a,b). Sterigmatocystin was shown to aerosolize from a finishing material (Moularat, Robine, 2008), at an airflow rate of 100 cm/s and a relative humidity of 30%. These studies demonstrate that mycotoxins are present in the indoor environment and that the levels may be higher in buildings affected by mould or damp. It is still not clear, however, whether the levels of airborne mycotoxins in damp buildings are sufficiently high to cause adverse health effects (see section 4.2.2).

2.3.6 Microbial and other volatile organic compounds

Several fungi produce volatile metabolites, which are a mixture of compounds that can be common to many species, although some also produce compounds that are genera- or species-specific. Microbial volatile organic compounds are often similar to common industrial chemicals. To date, more than 200 of these compounds derived from different fungi have been identified (Wilkins, Larsen, Simkus, 2000, 2003), including various alcohols, aldehydes, ketones, terpenes, esters, aromatic compounds, amines and sulfur-containing compounds. As few of those compounds are specific to fungi, measuring (microbial) volatile organic compounds is therefore of limited use in identifying indoor fungal growth. Detection of specific organic compounds does, however, permit a conclusion of fungal growth (visible or hidden), even if the results are not quantitative (Moularat et al., 2008a,b). No larger field studies have been conducted to compare mouldy and control buildings, and microbial volatile organic compounds have been measured only rarely in health surveys. Data on airborne concentrations are therefore scarce.

Some exposures with adverse health effects associated with damp indoor environments include emissions of volatile organic compounds from damp and mouldy building materials (Claeson, Sandstrom, Sunesson, 2007). Emissions are a consequence of competition between moisture and some chemicals for adsorption sites. Volatile organic compounds can be similar to microbial ones, as both often occur in the same environment. The main difference is the source of emission, i.e. mould or building materials. Damp concrete floors have been shown to increase chemical degradation of the plasticizer in polyvinyl chloride floor coatings and glues, resulting in emissions of volatile organic compounds such as 2-ethyl-1-hexanol (Norbäck et al., 2000; Tuomainen, Seuri, Sieppi, 2004). Similarly, damp concrete floors may emit ammonia from the self-levelling flooring compound used in the late 1970s and early 1980s in Europe. Furthermore, the offgassing of formaldehyde from composite wood products and the rate of formation of ozone increase with relative air humidity (Arundel et al., 1986; Godish, Rouch, 1986). Formaldehyde concentrations may also be elevated in damp indoor environments because moist air holds more formaldehyde. The levels of semi-volatile compounds, such as pentachlorophenol (a wood preservative) and other pesticides, may also be elevated in damp indoor environments. No studies have systematically addressed the link between levels of volatile organic compounds and dampness in indoor environments.

2.3.7 Viruses

It has been hypothesized that damp indoor environments with sufficiently high air humidity prolong the survival of respiratory viruses, so that the occupants are at greater risk of respiratory infection and, possibly, the onset of allergic disease (Hersoug, 2005). Although some experimental evidence shows significantly better survival times for several common cold-causing viruses, no real-life data are available. It is therefore unclear whether exposure to viruses should be considered as a risk associated with damp indoor spaces.

2.4   Exposure assessment

Exposure can be defined as an event during which people come into contact with a pollutant at a certain concentration during a certain length of time (WHO Regional Office for Europe, 2006a). In most circumstances, however, exposure defined in this way cannot be determined confidently, and exposure indicators are used instead. Thus, when the word exposure is used without qualification in this document, it refers to indicators. The indicators of exposure in indoor environments used most commonly are derived from answers to questionnaires. A more objective approach (but not necessarily a more valid one; see below) might be to measure the airborne or surface concentrations of indoor pollutants, such as the amount of pollutant per cubic metre of air or per gram of house dust. These are, however, generally relatively crude proxies of the true exposure and thus lead to at least some misclassification of exposure and subsequent bias.

The relative lack of knowledge about the role of specific exposures in health problems related to house dampness is due mainly to a lack of valid, quantitative methods for assessing exposure, particularly of bioaerosols. This may explain the relatively large number of studies that have failed to demonstrate a direct association between bioaerosol concentrations and health effects in damp indoor environments (see Chapter 4). This section discusses the issues of exposure assessment related to observed and perceived dampness and of bioaerosol measurements. Measurement of humidity in the air and of the moisture content of building materials is discussed in Chapter 3.

2.4.1 Measurement of indicators of dampness

Occupants' perceptions are the basis used for assessing house dampness in most epidemiological studies, and questionnaires are therefore often the method chosen. The questions typically elicit information on whether conditions such as leaks, flooding, wet basements, window condensation, visible fungal growth or mouldy odours are or have been present. Sometimes, the extent of water damage and damp is also assessed. Prevalence estimates may vary widely, however, depending on the way in which such questions are framed, the type of question, the level of detail requested and the judgement of the people filling in the questionnaire.

Reliance on self-reporting, which is by definition subjective, may be a source of error in cross-sectional studies, as demonstrated by Dales, Miller and McMullen (1997), who reported that under some conditions people with allergies are more likely than non-allergic people to report visible fungal growth. Other studies have shown that such bias is unlikely (Verhoeff et al., 1995; Zock et al., 2002). To overcome the problems associated with the bias of self-reporting, trained inspectors have been used in several studies to visit houses and assess indoor dampness, including its severity. This method has the advantage of being more objective and allows a more standardized approach; nevertheless, it is often a single snapshot, which lacks the longer perspective of the occupants. These differences in approaches may lead to different estimates of the prevalence of house dampness, as demonstrated in several comparisons of the two methods (see section 2.1).

Measurements of humidity in air, the moisture content of building materials, their interrelationships and their relationship with indoor climate dynamics more generally are discussed in Chapter 3.

2.4.2 Measurement of microorganisms and microbial agents

The assessment of indoor concentrations of microorganisms presents distinct challenges. Pathogenic microorganisms may be hazardous at extremely low levels, while other organisms may become important health hazards only at concentrations that are orders of magnitude higher. Some organisms and spores are extremely resilient, while others are inactivated during sampling. Certain fungal spores are easily identified and counted, while many bacteria are difficult to characterize. Sensitive, specific methods are available for quantifying some microbial agents, while there are no good methods for others. Many of the newly developed methods (e.g. measurement of microbial agents such as fungal $(1\rightarrow3)$-β-D-glucans or fungal extracellular polysaccharides; see below) have not been well validated and are often unavailable commercially. Even with some well-established methods (e.g. the *Limulus* amoebocyte lysate assay for measuring bacterial endotoxins; see below), significant variations in concentrations have been found (Thorne et al., 1997; Chun et al., 2000; Reynolds et al., 2002). Issues about the storage and transport of bioaerosol samples have often not been addressed, although these conditions can affect the activity of some biological agents, such as endotoxins (Thorne et al., 1994; Douwes et al., 1995; Duchaine et al., 2001). Furthermore, not all the biological agents that might be associated with damp indoor environments and their health effects may have been identified.

Most studies of dampness and health have focused on visible fungi or water damage, and in most of these studies exposure was assessed from questionnaires. The extent to which questionnaire reports of fungal growth correlate with actual exposure to relevant fungal components is, however, not known. In studies with objective measurements of fungal concentrations, spores were generally cultured from indoor air (Garrett et al., 1998) or from settled dust (Jacob et al., 2002). The section below gives the options available for measuring concentrations of micro-organisms (particularly fungi) in indoor air.

2.4.2.1. Culture-based methods

Airborne concentrations of microorganisms can be studied by counting cultur-able propagules in air samples or settled dust samples. Sampling of culturable microorganisms is based on impaction (in which microorganisms are collected from the airstream due to an inertial force that deposits them onto a solid or semisolid collection surface), liquid impingement (in which inertia as a princi-ple force collects microorganisms in a liquid medium) or air filtration (separa-tion of microorganisms from the airstream by passage through a porous medium such as a filter). After sample collection, colonies of bacteria and fungi are grown on culture media at a defined temperature for the length of time required for colony development (usually 3–7 days). Colonies are counted manually or by im-age analysis techniques. To date, no standard methods are available for detecting and enumerating fungi in indoor environments, which significantly limits the potential for comparing data from different studies. International standards are, however, being prepared by the International Organization for Standardization (ISO) technical committee 147/SC on indoor air for sampling by filtration and impaction and for the cultivation of fungi (ISO 16000-16, -17,-18).

Counting culturable microorganisms has some serious limitations. These in-clude poor reproducibility; selection of certain species because of, for example, the choice of sampling method, culture media or temperature chosen; and the lack of detection of non-culturable and dead microorganisms, cell debris and mi-crobial components, although they too may have toxic or allergenic properties. In addition, no good methods for sampling personal air for culturable micro-organisms are available, and air sampling for more than 15 minutes is often not possible, whereas air concentrations usually vary widely over time (see section 2.4.5). Nevertheless, counting culturable microorganisms is potentially a very sensitive technique, allowing the identification of many different species.

Traditional culture methods have proven to be of limited use for quantitative assessment of exposure. Culture-based techniques thus usually provide qualita-tive rather than quantitative data. The former can, however, be important in risk assessment, as not all fungal and bacterial species pose the same hazard. Further-more, a qualitative comparison of indoor and outdoor microbiota (in samples collected at the same time) may provide important information about potential indoor sources of contamination. More extensive reviews of techniques for sampling and culturing microorganisms are available (Eduard, Heederik, 1998; Macher, 1999).

2.4.2.2. Non-culture-based methods

In non-culture-based methods, organisms are enumerated regardless of their viability. Non-culturable microorganisms are generally sampled by air filtration or liquid impingement methods. Microorganisms can be stained with a fluorochrome, such as acridine orange, and counted under an epifluorescence microscope (Thorne et al., 1994).

Slit impaction on glass slides and staining with lactophenol blue is a common method for microscopic determination of the total concentration of fungal spores. The possibility of classifying microorganisms taxanomically is limited because little structure can be observed. Electron microscopy or scanning electron microscopy allows better determination (Eduard et al., 1988; Karlsson, Malmberg, 1989). Bacteria collected on impingers or filters can be counted by flow cytometry after staining with 4′,6-diamino-2-phenylindole or by fluorescent in situ hybridization (Lange, Thorne, Lynch, 1997).

The main advantage of microscopy and flow cytometry is that both culturable and non-culturable microorganisms can be quantified, selection effects are limited, personal air sampling is possible, the sampling time can – for many microorganisms – be varied over a wide range, and results are available quickly. The disadvantages include the unknown validity of these techniques, lack of detection of possibly relevant toxic or allergenic components or cell debris, limited possibilities for determining microorganisms, laborious and complicated procedures, and high cost per sample of the more advanced methods. An extensive review of microscopy and flow cytometry methods for counting nonculturable microorganism has been published (Eduard, Heederik, 1998). Little or no experience has been gained in non-industrial indoor environments with more advanced non-culture-based methods, such as scanning electron and epifluorescence microscopy and flow cytometry. Therefore the usefulness of these methods for indoor risk assessment is unknown.

2.4.2.3. Methods for assessing microbial constituents

Constituents or metabolites of microorganisms can be measured to estimate microbial exposure, instead of counting culturable or non-culturable microbial propagules. Toxic (e.g mycotoxins) or pro-inflammatory components (e.g endotoxins) can be measured, and non-toxic molecules can be used as markers of large groups of microorganisms or of specific microbial genera or species. The availability of methods, such as those based on the polymerase chain reaction (PCR) and immunoassays, has opened new avenues for detection and identification of species, regardless of whether the organisms are culturable.

Markers for the assessment of fungal biomass include ergosterol, measured by gas chromatography–mass spectrometry (Miller, Young, 1997), and fungal extracellular polysaccharides, measured in specific enzyme immunoas says (Douwes et al., 1999). These allow partial identification of the mould genera present. Volatile organic compounds produced by fungi, which may be suitable markers of fungal growth (Dillon, Heinsohn, Miller, 1996; Moularat et al., 2008b), are usually measured in air samples by gas chromatography with or without mass spectrometry or high-pressure liquid chromatography. Other agents, such as $(1\rightarrow3)$-β-D-glucans (Aketagawa et al., 1993; Douwes et al., 1996) and bacterial endotoxins, are measured because of their toxic potency. Endotoxins are measured with a *Limulus* amoebocyte lysate test, prepared from blood cells of the horseshoe crab, *Limulus polyphemus* (Bang, 1956). Analytical chemistry techniques with gas chromatography–mass spectrometry for quantifying lipopolysaccharides have also been developed (Sonesson et al., 1988, 1990); however, these methods require special extraction procedures and have not been widely used. Two methods for measuring $(1\rightarrow3)$-β-D-glucans have been described, one of which is based on the *Limulus* amoebocyte lysate assay (Aketagawa et al., 1993) and the other on an enzyme immunoassay (Douwes et al., 1996).

PCR techniques are available for the identification of species of bacteria and fungi in air (Alvarez et al., 1994; Khan, Cerniglia, 1994), and several quantitative PCR methods have been validated for use in the indoor environment. For example, real-time PCR methods have been described to detect and quantify *Cladosporium* (Zeng et al., 2006) and *Aspergillus* (Goebes et al., 2007) at the genus level. Similar methods have been developed for measuring species of common indoor fungi (Vesper et al., 2005; Meklin et al., 2007). PCR methods allow the assessment of large groups of microorganisms. For instance, a quantitative PCR method is available for measuring 36 indicator species commonly associated with damp houses in the United States and has been used to define an "environmental relative mouldiness index" for houses in that country (Vesper et al., 2007). PCR methods for quantitative assessment of exposure to fungi and other microorganisms have significant advantages, including sensitivity and specificity. Also, they can be used for quantitative assessment; they provide results relatively quickly; they can be used to measure a wide range of microorganisms, both genus and species; and they are independent of the culturability of the organism.

Most methods for measuring microbial constituents (with the exception of that for bacterial endotoxins) are experimental and have yet to be used routinely or are unavailable commercially. Important advantages of these methods include the stability of most of the measured components, allowing longer sampling times for airborne measurements and frozen storage of samples before analysis; the use of standards in most of the methods; and the possibility of testing for reproducibility. These methods do not, however, leave fungal isolates for further investigation.

2.4.3   Measurement of indoor allergens

Antibody-based immunoassays, particularly enzyme-linked immunosorbent assays, are widely used to measure aeroallergens and allergens in settled dust in buildings. These assays involve use of antibodies specific to the target allergen and an enzymic reaction with a substrate for detection. In radioimmunoassays, radiolabelling is used for detection. The house dust mite allergens Der p I, Der f I and Der p/f II have been widely investigated and the methods well described (Luczynska et al., 1989; Price et al., 1990; Leaderer et al., 2002). Methods for assessing exposure to allergens from rodents (Swanson, Agarwal, Reed, 1985; Schou, Svendson, Lowenstein, 1991; Hollander, Heederik, Doekes, 1997), cockroaches (Pollart et al., 1994) and storage mites (Iversen et al., 1990) have been published.

Methods for measuring fungal allergens are not widely available, mainly because of difficulties in manufacturing and standardizing fungal allergen extracts (see section 2.3.1). Nonetheless, some enzyme-linked immunosorbent assays have been described in the literature, and a commercial assay is available for *A. alternata* allergen (Alt a I). A comparison of several monoclonal and polyclonal antibody-based assays for measuring Alt a I (including a commercially available method) showed, however, wide disparity (Barnes et al., 2006). It is therefore unclear whether these assays provide valid estimates of the true *Alternaria* allergen concentrations in indoor samples.

2.4.4   Strategies for monitoring exposure

In addition to questionnaires, personal or environmental monitoring is commonly used for exposure assessment. Although monitoring can potentially result in a more valid, accurate assessment, this may not always be the case. Validity is strongly dependent on the sampling strategy chosen, which in turn depends on a large number of factors, including: the type of exposure and disease or symptoms of interest; whether the health outcomes are acute or chronic (e.g. exacerbation versus development of disease); whether the approach is population- or patient-based; suspected variations in exposure over both time and space and between diseased and reference populations; the methods available to assess exposure; and the costs of sampling and analysis.

2.4.4.1. What should be measured?

With regard to health problems associated with indoor air, many exposures should be considered, as it is often unclear which microorganisms or agents are causing the symptoms or diseases. Some studies are conducted specifically to assess which exposures are contributing to the development of symptoms. In practice, both funding and the availability of methods for measuring agents are limited, as many methods are not commercially available and are used only in research, severely limiting the possibility of measuring all agents of interest.

2.4.4.2. How useful are routinely collected data?

Data collected for use in monitoring may be of limited value in epidemiological studies. For example, monitoring is often done in areas where the concentrations are likely to be highest, to ensure compliance with exposure limits. In contrast, epidemiological studies require information on average concentrations. Special surveys may therefore be necessary, with random sampling, rather than relying on data collected during monitoring.

2.4.4.3. When should sampling be done?

To the extent possible, samples should be taken so that they represent the true exposure at an appropriate time. For acute effects, exposure measured shortly before the effects occur is the most useful. The situation is more complicated for chronic effects, as, ideally, exposure should be assessed before the effects occur and preferably at the time they are biologically most relevant – that is, when the exposure is considered the most problematic or when people are most likely to be exposed. This is possible only in prospective cohort studies or in retrospective cohort studies in which information on past exposure is available; even then, it is often unclear when people are most likely to be exposed to the agent of interest. In cross-sectional studies, exposure measurement can be valuable for assessing past exposure, but only when the environment has not changed significantly.

2.4.4.4. How many samples should be taken?

Measures of exposure should be sufficiently accurate and precise that the effect on disease can be estimated with minimal bias and maximum efficiency. Precision can be gained (i.e. measurement error can be reduced) by increasing the number of samples taken, either by increasing the number of people for whom exposure is measured or by increasing the number of measurements per person. In population studies, repeated sampling is particularly effective for exposures known to vary more widely over time within people than among people. If the within-people variation is lower than that between people, repeated measurements will not reduce the measurement error significantly. If there is known within- and between-person variation (from previous surveys or pilot studies, for example), the number of samples required to reduce bias in the risk estimate by a specific amount can be computed in the manner described by Cochran (1968) (see also section 2.4.5).

2.4.4.5. Should settled dust or airborne samples be taken?

In many studies, reservoir dust from carpets or mattresses is collected, and the concentrations are usually expressed in either weight per gram of sampled dust or weight per square metre. Although both measures are generally accepted, the latter may better reflect actual exposure (Institute of Medicine, 2004). The advantage of settled dust sampling is the presumed integration over time that occurs in deposition of the pollutant on surfaces (Institute of Medicine, 2000). Microorganisms can also proliferate in carpets, provided there is sufficient access to water; however, surface samples allow only a crude measure that is probably only a poor surrogate for airborne concentrations.

Airborne sampling requires very sensitive analytical methods. In addition, for an accurate assessment, large numbers of samples must be collected, as the temporal variation in airborne concentrations is probably very high (see section 2.4.5). Airborne sampling after agitation of settled dust has been used in some studies (Rylander et al., 1992, 1998; Rylander, 1997b; Thorn, Rylander, 1998), but it is questionable whether this results in a more valid exposure assessment. Therefore, exposure assessment is generally uncertain and this may obscure exposure–response relationships in epidemiological studies.

The recently described dustfall collector, a simple passive tool for long-term collection of airborne dust, combines the two methods to some extent (Würtz et al., 2005). Collectors are placed on shelves or cupboards at least 1.5 m above the floor and receive airborne dust by sedimentation; they can be used for up to several months. This method is not affected by short-term temporal variance in airborne concentrations and is probably a better surrogate for airborne exposures relevant to indoor health. The dustfall collector is cheap to produce and simple to use, and the microbial levels measured with this device appear to correlate with the degree of moisture in school buildings. Although the initial results look promising, more validation is required to assess the usefulness of the device for measuring indoor exposure.

2.4.4.6. Should ambient or personal airborne sampling be conducted?

In general, personal measurements best represent the risk of the relevant exposure, and personal sampling is therefore preferred to area sampling. Modern sampling equipment is now sufficiently light and small that it can be used for personal sampling, and several studies of chemical air pollution have demonstrated its feasibility both indoors and outdoors (Janssen et al., 1999, 2000). Personal sampling might not always be possible, however, for practical reasons, such as being too cumbersome for the study participants or a lack of portable equipment for making the desired measurements (of viable microorganisms, for example). Nonetheless, it is expected that greater use of new, sensitive exposure assessment methods, including quantitative PCR techniques to measure indoor microbial concentrations (see section 2.4.2), will overcome some of these constraints, in particular when used in combination with passive personal samplers.

2.4.5   Problems in measuring indoor exposure

Exposure to microorganisms in the indoor environment is most frequently assessed by counting culturable spores in settled dust or the air, but this approach has serious drawbacks (see section 2.4.2). Perhaps the most important problem, which has rarely been acknowledged in the literature, is that air sampling for more than 15 minutes is often not possible, since air concentrations usually vary a great deal over time. The few studies in which repeated measurements were made of fungi in air or in settled dust showed considerable temporal variation in concentrations, even over short periods (Hunter et al., 1988; Verhoeff et al., 1994b). The variation in the concentrations of isolated genera was even more substantial (Verhoeff et al., 1994b; Chew et al., 2001).

It has been suggested that in order to achieve a ratio of 3–4 for within- and between-house variation in concentration, which appears to be realistic for culturable indoor fungi (Verhoeff et al., 1994b), 27–36 samples should be taken per house. This is necessary for reliable estimates of the average concentration in an epidemiological study with less than 10% bias in the relationship between a health end-point and the exposure (Heederik, Attfield, 2000; Heederik et al., 2003).

Thus, unless many samples are taken per house, sampling of culturable organisms will probably result in a poor quantitative measure of exposure, leading to a nonspecific bias towards the null. This might explain why most studies that included measurements of culturable fungi found no association with symptoms (in contrast to reported mould). The issue is particularly relevant for measurements of viable microorganisms; nonetheless, similar problems may exist for airborne measurements of other bioaerosols, such as house dust mite allergens, endotoxins and fungal $(1{\rightarrow}3)$-β-D-glucans, as the airborne concentrations of these agents are also likely to be characterized by high temporal variation. This problem can be overcome by increasing the sampling time (up to several days or weeks), which is feasible for most bioaerosols, except viable microorganisms. This is often considered to be impractical, and therefore most exposure measurements continue to involve surface sampling, which is generally less affected by temporal variation. Surface sampling, however, may be a poor proxy for airborne concentrations (see above).

As no health-based exposure limits for indoor biological agents have been recommended, interpretation of concentrations is difficult, particularly in case studies. Therefore, strategies to evaluate indoor concentrations (either quantitatively or qualitatively) should include comparisons of exposure data with background levels or, better, comparisons of the exposure levels of symptomatic and non-symptomatic persons or in damp and non-damp buildings. A quantitative evaluation involves comparisons of concentrations, whereas a qualitative evaluation could consist of comparisons of species or genera of microorganisms in different environments. Because of differences in climatic and meteorological conditions and in the measurement protocols used in different studies (e.g. viable or non-viable sampling or by type of sampler or analysis), reference material in the literature can seldom be used.

2.5   Summary and conclusions

The prevalence of indoor damp is estimated to be in the order of 10–50%. It is highest in deprived neighbourhoods, where it often significantly exceeds the national average. Many case reports have also shown dampness and mould problems in office buildings, schools and day-care centres, but it is unclear what proportion of these buildings is affected. High air humidity, condensation and water damage promote the survival and growth of dust mites and fungi, resulting in increased exposure to mite and fungal allergens and fungal toxins and irritants. Damp indoor environments may also contain bacteria, bacterial endotoxins and other microorganisms, such as amoeba, but less information is available about these agents and further research is required. Damp building materials may increase their chemical degradation, resulting in more emissions of volatile organic compounds, including formaldehyde, further deterioration of building materials and structural integrity and subsequent use (and misuse) of potentially hazardous chemicals such as pesticides. Although it is plausible that the exposures listed above are the main causal factors of the health effects associated with damp buildings, this has not been proven.

Risk assessment is seriously hampered by a lack of valid methods for quantitative assessment of exposure. The usual culture methods for quantifying exposure to microbes have major limitations. Non-culture methods for assessing microbial constituents (e.g. microbial DNA, allergens, endotoxins, $(1{\rightarrow}3)$-β-D-glucans and fungal extracellular polysaccharides) appear more promising, although experience with these methods is generally limited. Therefore, more research is needed to establish better exposure assessment tools, and newly developed methods must undergo rigorous validation.

If exposure in indoor environments is to be monitored and valid conclusions are to be drawn, it is important also to include measurements of people without symptoms and measurements in buildings without damp. Furthermore, interpretation of airborne sampling should be based on multiple samples, as space–time variation in the environment is high. Proper interpretation of indoor measurements also requires detailed information about sampling and analytical procedures (including quality control) and awareness of the problems associated with these procedures. If methods for culturable organisms are used, comparisons with outdoor microbiota might provide further qualitative evidence of potential indoor sources of contamination.

3. Moisture control and ventilation

Olli Seppänen and Jarek Kurnitski

3.1 Introduction

Buildings provide shelter from climate for their occupants. Local resources, culture, climate and building traditions have significant effects on building design and construction. Since buildings have long lifetimes and use a significant portion of national assets, the construction industry is regulated by international or national codes and guidelines. Building codes are usually intended to ensure the quality of buildings: their safety and health properties and also the sustainable use of natural resources, such as energy, to reduce the environmental impact of the built environment. With increasing scientific understanding of the problems represented by moisture and dampness and recognition of the widespread nature of these problems, all countries must pay proper attention to how the quality of construction affects these problems. As construction practices vary among countries, it is difficult to create guidelines that are applicable in all regions. Nevertheless, many problems have the same origin and their solutions are thus similar in principle. The purpose of this chapter is to characterize the sources of and solutions for moisture and dampness problems in buildings and discuss the role of ventilation in controlling moisture and providing a healthy indoor environment.

Ventilation is intended to remove or dilute pollutants and to control the thermal environment and humidity in buildings. It must be sufficient either to remove pollutants and humidity generated indoors or to dilute their concentrations to acceptable levels for the health and comfort of the occupants and must be sufficient to maintain the building's integrity. A number of reviews (Seppänen, Fisk, Mendell, 1999; Wargocki et al., 2002, Sundell, Levin, 2007) have shown an association between ventilation and health, although the precise exposure–response relationship differs by study. As exact values for ventilation cannot be identified and limit values have not been set for all pollutants, it is seldom possible to determine the necessary ventilation rates and the associated risks on the basis of pollutant concentrations. Selection of ventilation rates is based on epidemiological research, laboratory and field experiments, odour perception, irritation, occupant preferences, productivity, and experience.

Ventilation can be provided by various natural and mechanical methods. These usually improve health but may also have adverse effects (Seppänen, Fisk, 2002; Wargocki et al., 2002) if not properly designed, installed, maintained and operated (Mendell, Smith 1990; Seppänen, 2004; Mendell et al., 2007), as ventilation can then allow the entry of harmful substances that degrade the indoor environment. Ventilation also affects air and moisture flow through the building envelope and may therefore lead to moisture problems that degrade the structure. Ventilation changes pressure differences across a building and may cause or prevent the infiltration of pollutants from building structures or adjacent spaces. While ventilation is used to control humidity, under certain circumstances it can result in very high or very low humidity. Humidity is an important parameter when considering limiting the use of outdoor air ventilation.

In non-residential buildings and in hot climates, ventilation is often integrated with air-conditioning, which complicates the operation of these systems. The addition of humidifiers to ventilation systems or as stand-alone units can introduce excess humidity, chemicals (used to treat the water in humidification systems) or microorganisms that grow on components in humid locations, such as drip pans in air-conditioning units or humidifiers.

In some studies, the prevalence of symptoms of the sick-building syndrome has been associated with the characteristics of the heating, ventilation and air-conditioning system. On average, the prevalence of such symptoms was higher in air-conditioned than in naturally ventilated buildings, independent of humidification (Mendell, Smith, 1990; Seppänen, Fisk, 2002). The evidence suggests that better hygiene, commissioning, operation and maintenance of air-handling systems is particularly important in reducing the negative effects of heating, ventilation and air-conditioning systems (Mendell, Smith, 1990; Sieber et al., 1996; Seppänen, Fisk, Mendell, 1999; Mendell et al., 2003, 2006, 2008). Thus, moisture and microbial contamination – not only in the building structure or surfaces, but also in heating, ventilation and air-conditioning systems – has adverse health effects.

Exposure to pollutants in indoor air generated by indoor activities and emitted from indoor materials or ventilation systems can have a variety of effects with a broad range of severity, from the perception of unwanted odours to cancer (e.g. from radon). The effects can be acute or longer-term. The positive and negative effects of ventilation and ventilation systems include the following (European Collaborative Action on Urban Air, Indoor Environment and Human Health, 2003; Seppänen, Fisk, 2004).

- Ventilation dilutes the concentrations of (or disperses) airborne viruses or bacteria that can cause infectious diseases. Thus, higher ventilation rates reduce the prevalence of airborne infectious diseases (Fisk at al., 2002; Li Y et al., 2007).
- Some microorganisms can grow in cooling-coils and drip pans, as well as air humidifiers and cooling towers, thus causing respiratory diseases or symptoms, such as legionnaires disease and humidifier fever (Flannigan, Morey, 1996). Further evidence was provided by a blinded intervention study that

showed significant reductions in respiratory and other symptoms during periods of ultraviolet irradiation of coils and pans in office buildings (Menzies et al., 2003).

- Ventilation rates below 10 l/s per person are associated with significantly higher prevalences of one or more health outcomes or with worse perceived air quality in office environments (Seppänen, Fisk, Mendell, 1999).
- Ventilation rates greater than 10 l/s per person, up to approximately 20–25 l/s per person, are associated with a significant decrease in the prevalence of symptoms of sick-building syndrome or with improved perceived air quality in office environments (Seppänen, Fisk, Mendell, 1999; Sundell, Levin, 2007).
- Improved ventilation can improve task performance and productivity in the office environment (Seppänen, Fisk, Lei, 2006).
- Ventilation rates below half an air change per hour are a health risk in Nordic residential buildings (Wargocki et al., 2002; Sundell, Levin, 2007).
- Ventilation rates up to 9 l/s per pupil in schools improve performance in school tasks (Wargocki, Wyon, 2006a,b).
- In comparison with natural ventilation, air-conditioning (with or without humidification) is often associated with a statistically significant increase in the prevalence of one or more sick-building syndrome symptoms in office buildings (Seppänen, Fisk, 2002).
- Indoor humidity is influenced by ventilation rates. Ventilation usually reduces indoor moisture levels. Very high indoor humidity is associated with increased growth of microorganisms such as mould and bacteria (Institute of Medicine, 2004).
- Relative humidity greater than approximately 50% increases indoor dust mite levels. Low ventilation rates may thus increase the prevalence or intensity of allergic and other symptoms (Flannigan, Morey, 1996).
- Pathogenic microorganisms can be transported by ventilation systems, and some evidence indicates that inadequate ventilation rates in general hospital rooms influence exposure to airborne infectious agents, such as tubercle bacilli (Menzies et al., 2000). Insufficient information is available, however, to specify minimum ventilation requirements for hospitals, schools and offices in relation to the spread of airborne infectious diseases (Li Y et al., 2007).
- Increased risks of lung cancer, heart attack, heart disease and stroke have been linked to exposure to environmental tobacco smoke and to radon decay products. Ventilation rates usually reduce the indoor concentrations of these agents.

The characteristics of ventilation include the rate, the type of system, the contaminants in indoor air and the physical characteristics of the indoor environment. These characteristics affect human responses individually and collectively. Also, ventilation can affect other aspects of the indoor environment that in turn affect health, including thermal conditions, indoor humidity, pressure differences across the building envelope, draught and noise.

The relationships between absolute humidity (moisture content of the air, measured in grams of water per kilogram of dry air), temperature and relative humidity are shown in Figure 2, where the relative humidity of air is presented as curves, temperature is on the vertical axis and the absolute humidity on the horizontal axis. The following are examples of how relative humidity is affected by temperature, i.e. heating.

- When outdoor air at a temperature of –8 °C and 100% relative humidity, which is usually very high in winter (point A in Figure 2), is brought to an indoor temperature of 20 °C, its relative humidity decreases to 15%. Thus, cold outdoor air used in ventilation is effective in carrying moisture from indoors.
- When air at a temperature of 15 °C and an absolute humidity of 5.5 g of water in 1 kg of dry air (corresponding to a relative humidity of 50%) is heated to a temperature of 18 °C, its relative humidity decreases to 40%. Thus, heating can help to prevent high relative humidity.
- When air at a temperature of 20 °C and a relative humidity of 58% (point B in Figure 2) is cooled to 15 °C, its relative humidity increases to 75%; when the temperature is decreased to 11 °C, the relative humidity reaches 100%. Water condenses on surfaces at such temperatures. Thus, when the temperature in houses decreases locally (e.g. at window panes, unheated sections of the house or poorly insulated walls), the relative humidity rises and accelerates microbial growth.

3.2   Sources of moisture

Moisture has become a major cause of building damage: it has been estimated (Bomberg, Brown, 1993; Ronald, 1994) that 75–80% of all the problems with building envelopes are caused to a certain extent by moisture. Haverinen (2002) conducted cross-sectional analyses in the Finnish housing stock and found that 38% of detached houses and 25% of apartments had notable or significant moisture problems. A study of 420 buildings in Sweden (Wessén, Honkanen, Mälarstig, 2002) showed that moisture problems, resulting in vivid microbial growth with microbial or chemical emissions from building materials and microbial metabolites, were present in 65% of the buildings. The presence of house dampness or mould (i.e. damp spots, visible mould or mildew, water damage and flooding) was reported by 38% of participants in a Canadian study (Dales, Burnett, Zwanenburg, 1991). These estimates show that moisture problems are a serious issue. They also have a strong economic effect, as repair of extensive problems is expensive. Pirinen et al. (2005) estimated that the cost of repairing microbiological damage that resulted in adverse health effects in Finland was €10 000–40 000 per case.

Figure 2. Psychometric chart of relations between air temperature, absolute humidity (water in grams per kilogram of dry air) and relative humidity in the air

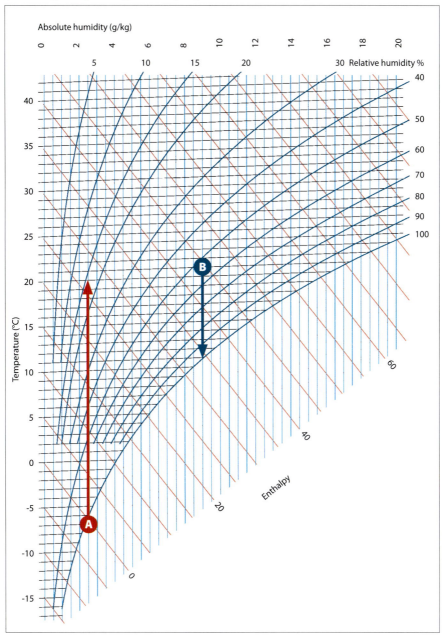

Phenomena related to water intrusion, dampness and excess moisture are not only harmful to the health of a building's occupants, but they also seriously affect the condition of the building structure, which may diminish the indoor air quality of the building.

In addition to the risks of wooden structures rotting and microbial growth, building materials may also be degraded by chemical processes induced by moisture. For example, installation of hard surface flooring or even textile carpets over concrete that is not sufficiently cured and therefore still has excess moisture can result in chemical reactions that produce alcohols and other volatile organic compounds. Flooring is often installed before the concrete is sufficiently dry, because of pressure to complete a construction quickly.

In a study of moisture problems in 291 Finnish houses, Pirinen (2006) found that about two thirds of moisture problems could be found by non-destructive methods, such as careful visual inspection. The remaining third were hidden in the structures and required comprehensive investigations with destructive methods, such as drilling holes, opening structures or taking material samples. Rainwater or groundwater or plumbing leaks and dampness caused by capillary suction were the commonest causes of the problems; however, a detailed technical examination showed a wide variety of 82 mechanisms.

Examples of the commonest moisture-related problems in buildings are:

- rainwater or groundwater leaking into the enclosure (roof, walls, windows or foundation), often resulting in mould growth, peeling paint, wood decay or corrosion;
- plumbing leaks and spills, perhaps resulting from improper design, installation, operation or maintenance (e.g. failure to inspect and repair plumbing leaks);
- water wicking (capillary suction) through porous building materials (such as concrete or wood) from a moisture source (such as rainwater or plumbing water) to a material that does not tolerate wetting;
- rainwater, condensation or plumbing water running along the top or bottom of a material (bridging), for example, along the top for some distance or clinging to the bottom of a truss, rafter, I-beam, floor joist or suspended ceiling track before falling or being absorbed by a porous material;
- infiltration of warm, moist outside air through cracks and holes in the enclosure during warm, humid weather – which can cause condensation on materials that are cooler, because they are part of the air-conditioning system – have been cooled by air-conditioned indoor air or are in cool basements or crawl spaces;
- exfiltration of warm, moist indoor air through cracks and holes in the enclosure during cold weather, which can cause condensation in wall and ceiling cavities and attic spaces;
- intentional or accidental vapour barriers in the wrong place, which can lead to condensation in the building enclosure;
- unvented or poorly vented sources, such as swimming pools, spas, aquariums, dishwashers, combustion devices, kitchens and baths, from which water

may condense in the building enclosure or, if indoor humidity levels are high enough, on materials in the space itself (e.g. ceilings, walls, furniture, cold-water pipes or air-conditioning air supply diffusers);

- insufficient dehumidification by heating, ventilating and air-conditioning systems, which may result in levels of interior humidity that are high enough to cause mould to grow on furniture, walls, ceilings or air-conditioning supply diffusers;
- poor condensate drainage due to heating, ventilation and air-conditioning system deficiencies; condensation from cooling coils may overflow drain pans or leak from condensate drain lines; and
- enclosure of wet materials in building assemblies during construction by materials that are prone to moisture problems and grow mould, delaminate or do not cure properly.

The technical causes of failure to control water damage, dampness or moisture are often closely connected to the climate. The prevailing temperature, humidity, rain and wind conditions regulate much of the principles and practices of construction, such as the foundation, insulation, structure of the building envelope and ventilation system. Indoor humidity is also physically connected to the outdoor climatic conditions. Therefore, the problems of building moisture and dampness, microbial contamination, repair and control vary with the climatic zone. Nevertheless, regardless of the climate, the prevention and control of moisture problems and their subsequent effects should be addressed in the early phases of building construction and in sustained maintenance of a building. Methods for controlling moisture are discussed in section 3.9.

3.3 Mould and mites as indicators of building performance

Measures can be taken to prevent mould, even though all the mechanisms by which microbial growth affects health are yet unknown. As described in section 2.2, the primary factor in the control of mould growth is moisture, especially relative humidity indoors and in structures. (Note that relative humidity above the substrate is the same as water activity, which is often used to describe mould growth conditions.)

The presence of mould and mites in a building is associated with the relative humidity of indoor air. As noted in section 2.2, mites require a relative humidity in excess of 45–50%. Therefore, to prevent the multiplication of dust mites in houses, the relative humidity during the heating season should be below this value.

Indoor relative humidity can be readily controlled by ventilation or air conditioning (see sections 3.4 and 3.8), by keeping it below the limit values for mould growth or mites. Even under such conditions, however, relative humidity can be higher on colder internal surfaces. This should be avoided by relevant hygrothermal design, which includes heat and moisture transfer analyses, application of the necessary thermal insulation and avoidance of thermal bridges. Relative humidity is much more difficult to control in structures than in indoor air as it is often dominated by outer climatic factors. Close consideration must be given to the hygrothermal performance of building assemblies, including mould growth, for the prevention of mould and moisture problems. Limit values for relative humidity on surfaces and structures and the mould growth models described in this chapter should be applied in the design of new buildings, in repairs and in field investigations of existing buildings, following the principles of hygrothermal design.

Even if the lowest relative humidity for germination of some species of fungi is 62–65%, experiments on common building and finishing materials indicate that susceptible surfaces can be kept free of fungal growth if the relative humidity is maintained below 75–80%. Mould fungi do not grow below a relative humidity of 80% (Adan, 1994) or below 75% within a temperature range of 5–40 °C (Viitanen, Ritschkoff, 1991).

After an extensive analysis of published data on laboratory experiments, Rowan et al. (1999) recommended that the relative humidity be maintained below 75% to limit fungal growth in buildings. Johansson et al. (2005), after a review of the literature, described the material-specific critical moisture conditions for microbiological growth: the critical relative humidity (maximum long-term relative humidity allowed for non-growth) was 75–90% for clean materials and 75–80% for contaminated or soiled materials (Table 2).

In reality, relative humidity and temperature on surfaces and in building structures change all the time, and mould formation is a time-dependent process that can be described by relative humidity, temperature and building material. Obviously, the relative humidity of the outdoor climate does not permit the relative humidity in building

Table 2. Critical relative humidity for various groups of materials

Material group	Relative humidity (%)
Wood and wood-based materials	75–80
Paper on plasterboard	80–85
Mineral insulation materials	90–95
Extruded and expanded polystyrene	90–95
Concrete	90–95

Source: Johansson et al. (2005).

structures to be kept below 75–80%. Therefore, a single limit value is inadequate for the hygrothermal design of building structures. In order to describe mould growth formation, dynamic models are needed that can take into account fluctuations in relative humidity and the time required for mould growth on a given material. To assess dynamic mould formation, dynamic data are required on the relative humidity and temperature in the structure or material studied, which can be either measured or calculated with simulation tools.

Viitanen et al. (2000) provided a differential equation (Eq. 1) for varying temperature and humidity conditions of pine and spruce. The equation (and the model based on it) predicts mould growth from an index, M, that varies between 0 and 6. A value of 0 indicates no mould growth; 1 indicates that some growth can be detected under a microscope, 3 that some mould growth can be detected visually, and 6 that very heavy, dense mould growth covers nearly 100% of the surface. The model takes into account temperature, surface relative humidity, the type of wood and the quality of the wood surface; it can also account for delay in mould growth due to temporarily low relative humidity. Equation 1 is as follows:

$$\frac{dM}{dt} = \frac{1}{7 \cdot \exp(-0.68\ln T - 13.9\ln RH + 0.14W - 0.33SQ + 66.02)} k_1 k_2 \quad \text{(Eq. 1)}$$

where M is the mould growth index, t is time calculated in days, T is temperature (0.1–40 °C), RH is relative humidity (%), W is the wood species (pine = 0, spruce = 1) and SQ is a factor that describes the quality of the wood surface (a resawn surface after drying = 0, a kiln-dried surface = 1). The coefficients k_1 and k_2 define the growth rate under favourable conditions and the upper limit of the mould growth index. This model is useful for analysing wooden building structures; however, it can be used only if the value of the mould growth index to be used as a design criterion has already been decided. Arguably, a mould growth index of 1 (some growth can be detected under a microscope) would be the relevant choice in most cases.

Another widely used mould growth model, which is applicable to many materials, is the isopleth model and its extension, the transient biohygrothermal model (Krus, Sedlbauer, 2007). Isopleths show the mould growth rate and the lowest boundary lines of possible fungus activity (lowest isopleth for mould). Isopleths are given for three categories of substrates (Figure 3), which differ in the availability of nutrients for fungi. The common building materials belong to categories 1 and 2. If we consider only the fungi that are discussed in the literature, because of their possible health effects (e.g. *A. fumigatus*, *A. flavus* and *S. chartarum*), the lowest isopleth for mould is slightly higher than that given in Figure 3 (Krus, Sedlbauer, 2002).

By use of the germination time and growth rate, the isopleth model allows an assessment of mould growth similar to that allowed by the model of Viitanen et al. (2000). Application of the isopleth model indicates the degree of germination (between 0 and 1) and growth in millimetres per day when the degree is one. The biohygrothermal model (Sedlbauer, 2001) allows an even more accurate assessment of mould growth, as it describes moisture transfer at the spore level, thus taking into account interim drying of fungal spores during transient microclimatic boundary conditions. Application of this model also gives mould growth in millimetres. The disadvantages of the isopleth models are that they can

Figure 3. Isopleth systems for three categories of substrate to determine the influence of the substrate on the formation of mould

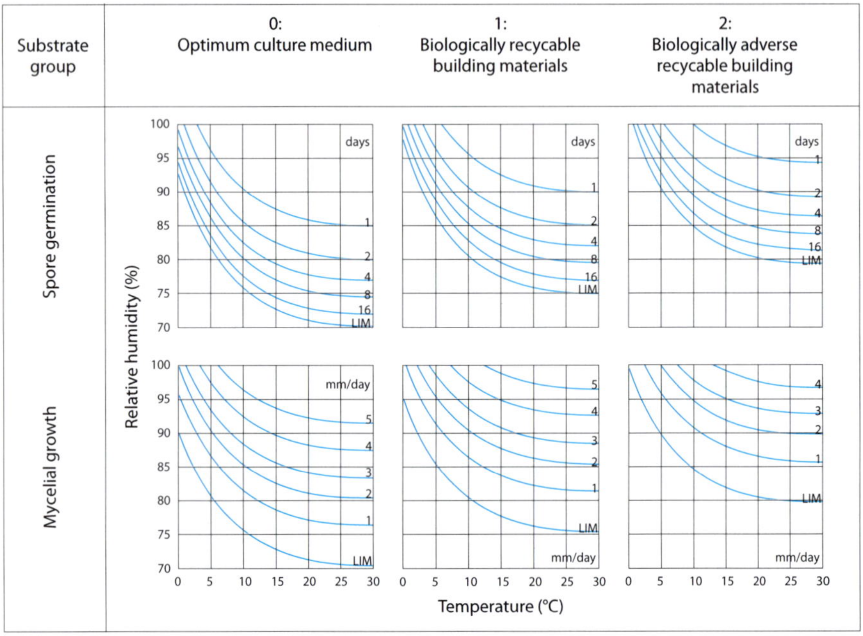

Source: Adapted from Sedlbauer *(2001).*
Note. days, germination time in days; mm/day, germination rate; LIM, lowest isopleth for mould for each substrate group.

be used only for assessing cumulative mould growth and do not allow assessment of mould growth decrement (as in the model of Viitanen et al.) when conditions became dry.

Dynamic mould growth models are very useful in assessing the hygrothermal performance of building assemblies. Predicted mould growth also correlates reasonably well with measured concentrations of spores (Pasanen et al., 2001), but such correlations are limited and can be application-specific. Mould growth models can support field investigations when the spore concentrations of material samples are measured. The availability of predicted mould growth makes it possible to conclude whether the measured spore concentration is typical of the structure or material being studied or if it indicates some failure in moisture performance, such as accidental leaks.

The main challenge of field investigations is to decide which contaminated materials should be removed and which can be left in building assemblies with a reasonably low risk of indoor climate problems. Spore concentrations in material samples can be measured easily, and mould growth can be predicted, but little is known about how indoor concentrations can be predicted from these results, even when epidemiological indoor spore concentration guidelines are available. For example, a limit value of 500 CFU/m^3 for airborne fungal spores in indoor air in urban areas in winter is used in Finland (Ministry of Social Affairs and Health,

2003). This value was derived by comparing buildings with and without moisture problems; concentrations below 500 CFU/m³ were found to be typical in Finnish buildings without moisture problems in winter. This value would be a straight-forward guideline for design if a method of calculation existed. However only limited information is available on fungal spore transport – for example, pen-etration factors must be determined by laboratory measurements (Airaksinen et al., 2004a). Thus, in order to realize the possibilities of mould growth models fully, relevant methods for calculating fungal spore levels and indoor air target values should be available.

3.4   Ventilation performance

Ventilation (outdoor airflow into a building) must be adequate to remove and dilute pollutants and humidity generated indoors, although the first alternative for improving indoor air quality should be control of pollutant sources. Ventila-tion should be energy efficient and arranged so that it does not degrade indoor air quality or climate and does not cause any harm to the occupants or to the building. Ventilation rates should be based on pollution loads, moisture genera-tion and use of the building. To the extent possible, outdoor pollutants should be removed from the air before the air is brought inside the building.

The concentration of indoor air pollutants or moisture can be used to calcu-late the ventilation rate needed for dilution of the pollutants or moisture to an acceptable steady-state level. Removal of humidity generated indoors can be cal-culated for the steady state from Equation 2. The equation assumes that the con-centrations at different locations indoors are equal, that the indoor concentration equals the exhaust air concentration and that the moisture contents of the build-ing and the interior materials are in equilibrium. In the following equation:

$$q_{vSUP} = \frac{G}{v_{IDA} - v_{SUP}} \qquad \text{(Eq. 2)}$$

q_{vSUP} is the volume flow rate of supply air (in m³/s), G is the indoor moisture gen-eration in the room (in g/s), v_{IDA} is the moisture per volume of indoor air in the room (in g/m³) and v_{SUP} is the moisture per volume of supply (outdoor) air (in g/m³).

Ventilation removes humidity at a rate of $q_{vSUP} \times (v_{IDA} - v_{SUP})$. More humidity is obviously removed (ventilation is more effective) at low outdoor air humidity. As cold air contains less absolute humidity than warm air, humidity removal is most effective at low outdoor temperatures. In hot climates, the outdoor humidity may be higher than the indoor humidity. In such cases, ventilation brings in humidity, and humidity is usually removed by air-conditioning (condensation on a cooling coil).

While high indoor relative humidity is problematic in mild and hot climates, very low relative humidity may be a problem in a cold climate. In a cold climate, low outdoor humidity during winter combined with overheating may decrease the indoor relative humidity to levels that provoke skin symptoms and nasal dryness and congestion (Reinikainen, Jaakkola, 2003). Kalamees (2006) measured an average relative humidity during winter of 26% in 94 Finnish houses and 32% in 27 Estonian houses. Humidified indoor air imposes a serious vapour pressure load on the building envelope; in hot climates, a similar effect is caused by dehumidification.

All relevant pollutants should be checked to determine which are the most critical. As a rule, source control is preferable to ventilation. Equation 2 above is valid for a steady-state situation (default situation); it also assumes that all pollution generated in a room is carried out with the airflow: no other pollutant sinks are assumed to be present. When the emission period of moisture is short, the stationary equilibrium concentration may not be achieved, or the airflow can be reduced for a given maximum concentration.

Kalamees (2006) measured average indoor moisture generation rates of 5.9 kg/day per house and 1.9 kg/day per person in 101 Finnish houses. Indoor humidity was calculated with Equation 2 with reasonable accuracy from data on ventilation and standard moisture generation from people, pets, house plants, cooking, showering, saunas and drying clothing.

Usually, moisture generation indoors is not continuous or in a steady state but is intermittent. To take this into account, a dynamic calculation with relevant indoor humidity generation profiles and material data (including moisture buffering effects) is needed. Many simulation tools are available for such calculations. The capacity of building and interior materials to absorb and release moisture has a significant effect on indoor humidity fluctuations and may have consequences for moisture damage and dampness. Moisture buffering effects are especially strong at low ventilation rates (Kurnitski et al., 2007). The recent general trend has been towards buildings with significantly lower moisture capacity, and this, together with generally reduced ventilation rates, may affect the prevalence of dampness-related problems.

3.5   Ventilation systems

Ventilation systems can be classified as natural, mechanical or a mixture of the two.

3.5.1   Natural ventilation

Natural ventilation usually uses no fans to move the outdoor air into and out of a building. Thus, the ventilation rates in natural ventilation depend on the size and distribution of the openings in the building envelope and on the magnitude of the driving forces (pressure differences), which are the stack effect and wind pressure. The stack effect depends on the height of the building (stack) and the temperature difference between indoor and outdoor air. Wind pressure depends on wind speed and direction. As the forces for air movement depend on the weather conditions, the openings in the building envelope must be controlled according to the weather as well as to pollutant and moisture generation. If the indoor environment is conditioned, the energy used to heat, cool, humidify or dehumidify the ventilation air can be significant. Therefore, ventilation rates that are too high should be avoided. High ventilation rates are not a problem in climates where indoor environments are not conditioned.

In cold and hot climates, the configuration and size of openings are a significant aspect of ventilation design. As the weather fluctuates constantly, the challenge of designing natural ventilation is to harness forces determining air movement, so that the flow into a space is maintained at the desired rate.

Often the term *natural ventilation* is applied to buildings that are ventilated haphazardly by relying on the leakage (cracks or porosity of structures) of the building combined with window openings, which can result in poor comfort and uncontrolled heat loss. Natural ventilation needs careful design and construction in order to supply adequate ventilation rates, although the occupant will usually have to adjust the ventilation openings when necessary. Inadequate ventilation rates can lead to serious dampness and health problems and moisture damage. Like any other technical system, natural ventilation has advantages and disadvantages. Its advantages include:

- its suitability for many types of buildings in mild or moderate climates;
- the associated open window environment, which is popular, especially in pleasant locations and mild climates;
- high airflow rates for cooling and purging if there are enough openings;
- short periods of discomfort during periods of warm weather;
- no need to provide space for a ventilation plant;
- minimum maintenance;
- usually, a lower cost of installation and operation than that of mechanical ventilation; and
- the absence of fan or system noise.

The disadvantages of natural ventilation include its:

- lack of suitability for severe climates, where the ingress of very cold air causes discomfort, condensation and high energy loss;
- inadequate control over the ventilation rate, which can lead to poor indoor air quality and excessive heat loss;
- varying airflow rates and patterns of airflow;
- impracticality of fresh air delivery and air distribution in large, deep, multi-room buildings;
- inadequacy in cases of high heat gains;

BOX 2   Types of natural ventilation

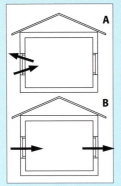

Single-sided ventilation (see diagram A) is the process by which air enters a building on the same side of a space as it leaves. Single-sided ventilation through a small opening is driven by random turbulent fluctuations of the pressure over the building facade. At best, this type of single-sided approach is unreliable and is not recommended as part of a controlled natural ventilation strategy.

Cross-flow ventilation (see diagram B) is the process by which air enters the building on one side of a space and leaves through an opening on the opposite side. Cross-flow designs form the basis of best practice in natural and hybrid ventilation systems. The pressure difference between the facades is influenced by wind, and it is typically much larger that the turbulent fluctuation in one facade; thus, adequate ventilation rates are easier to obtain and predict. Most controlled natural designs are based on cross flow. The system has limitations for ventilating deep-plan, multi-roomed buildings.

The wind tower consists of a vertical stack that, in cross-section, is divided into quadrants. In a space, the stack normally penetrates and terminates at ceiling level. Wind directed at the windward quadrant or quadrants is driven down the stack to ventilate the space below. Simultaneously, stale air is sucked out of the space, driven by the negative pressure generated by the wind on the leeward quadrant or quadrants. Such systems have been used in the desert regions of the Middle East for many centuries. Modern variants are used increasingly in locations where a strong wind driving force is available.

Stack systems consist of open vertical ducts that usually terminate at ceiling level in the ventilated space and, externally, just above roof level (Figure 5). In usual operation, warm air from the building exhausts from passive stacks, and make-up air is provided by room air vents or *trickle vents*. Stacks are usually used to promote extraction of air from *wet* rooms. Airflow is driven through the stack by a combination of stack pressure and wind-induced suction. Passive stacks are most suitable for moderate-to-medium cold climates, where there is a consistent winter driving force.

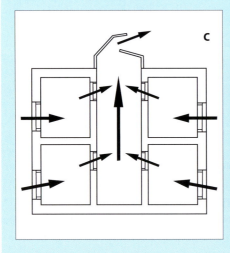

Atrium ventilation (see diagram C) uses a glass-covered courtyard (the atrium) which provides an all-weather space for the building occupants. It is popular for buildings such as offices and shopping malls and features *passive* low-energy building designs. Natural ventilation can be applied by using the atrium itself as a passive stack (see diagram C). In this case, the atrium is extended above the occupied zone by several metres to ensure that the *neutral pressure plane* is above the topmost occupied level. Flow patterns can be disrupted by wind-induced pressures. To adjust inaccessible top openings, automatic damper controls may be needed.

- unsuitability for noisy and polluted locations;
- security risk if ventilation depends mainly on openable windows;
- impracticality of heat recovery from exhaust air;
- obligation to adjust openings as necessary;
- inability to filter or clean incoming air;
- requirement for large-diameter ducts and restrictions on routing air in ducted systems; and
- increased occurrence of dampness and fungal growth in humid climates.

Various techniques or combinations of techniques are used to provide natural ventilation, including single-sided ventilation, cross-flow ventilation, wind towers, stack ventilation and atrium ventilation. They are described briefly in Box 2. In practice, controlled natural ventilation is best suited for buildings located in mild-to-moderate climates away from inner city locations. The buildings should be designed from the beginning for natural ventilation. This type of ventilation cannot be used in deep, multi-room buildings if it is constrained by climate and outside noise and pollution. The building types for which natural ventilation is suitable include dwellings (individual and apartments), small-to-medium-sized offices, schools, small-to-medium retail premises, recreational buildings, warehouses and industrial premises.

With natural ventilation, the required ventilation rate cannot be maintained in all weather conditions. Also, the building envelope cannot be made airtight, as is common practice in buildings with mechanical ventilation – to reduce energy losses due to infiltration and exfiltration. Figure 4 illustrates some of the problems related to natural ventilation systems that rely on temperature differences as a driving force. As the figure shows, under some weather conditions, pressure differences will reverse the airflow (blue arrows), and the exhaust air stacks, which may be contaminated, become supply routes and spread the pollutant into living rooms.

3.5.2 Mechanical ventilation

Mechanical ventilation is based on the requirement that the ventilation rate is maintained in all weather conditions without involving the occupants of the building. When ventilation is provided by a mechanical supply and exhaust system, the building envelope can be made airtight, and energy losses due to infiltration and exfiltration can therefore be reduced. A tight building envelope also improves sound insulation and reduces the transfer of external noise into the building. The energy efficiency of ventilation can be further improved through heat recovery from exhaust air, demand-controlled ventilation depending on occupancy, moisture or air quality factors. Air supplied for ventilation can be cleaned of outdoor air pollutants. Also, heating and cooling can easily be combined with mechanical ventilation systems. Moreover, mechanical ventilation systems may also control pressure differences over the building envelope and prevent moisture damage in building structures. It can be used in any type of building and allows freedom in architectural design, which may be the major reason for its rapid acceptance in modern building practice.

3.5.2.1. Mechanical exhaust ventilation

In mechanical exhaust ventilation systems, air is exhausted from rooms with greater pollutant generation and lower air quality. Air infiltration through the building envelope brings outdoor air for ventilation into the building. In apartment buildings, exhaust from the different floors can be connected to the same duct (Figure 5) if the pressure drop in the exhaust grille is high enough to prevent airflow from floor to floor. A central fan serves all the apartments. Room airflow can be controlled by adjustable grilles, according to humidity or the concentration of carbon dioxide or other pollutants, or by occupancy sensors.

The advantages of mechanical exhaust ventilation are a constant ventilation rate and the small negative pressure in the building, which prevents moisture migration into external walls and prevents condensation and (consequently) mould growth. It has several disadvantages, however. Air infiltrates through the building envelope, which creates draughts in winter in cold climates. Also, it is difficult to recover heat from exhaust air, and recovered heat cannot be used to heat ventilation air, although it can be used to preheat domestic hot water with a heat

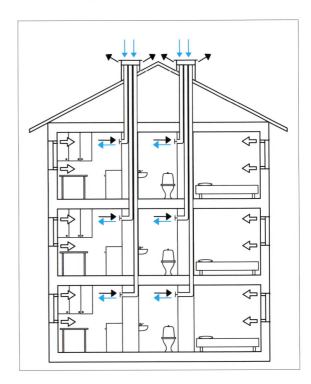

Figure 4. Under some weather conditions, the flow in the stack may be reversed (blue arrows) in natural ventilation systems that rely on temperature differences as a driving force

pump. As the exhaust usually comes from kitchens and bathrooms, the ventilation supply airflow is not evenly distributed in the bedrooms and living rooms. Furthermore, the distribution of outdoor air for ventilation depends on leakage in the building envelope.

3.5.2.2. Mechanical supply and exhaust ventilation

In mechanical supply and exhaust systems, the air is supplied via ducts and fans to bedrooms and living rooms in residential buildings and typically exhausted from kitchens, bathrooms and bedrooms. In other types of buildings, it is supplied to all occupied spaces. Exhaust air may flow through a heat exchanger before it is discharged outdoors. In the heat exchanger, a major part of the heat is recovered and used to heat the outdoor air for ventilation. This is usually the most economical use of recovered heat, as the need for heating is met by the available heat. Another use of recovered heat is for domestic hot water.

In an apartment building, a mechanical supply and exhaust system can be centralized (Figure 6) or decentralized For heat recovery to be beneficial, the heat recovered must exceed the additional energy expended by the fans. Where carbon is the basis for comparison and where the unit-embodied carbon is higher for electricity than for the primary heating fuel source (e.g. natural gas), its use in a moderate climate might be difficult to justify without a carefully designed ductwork system, an efficient heat exchanger and energy-efficient fans and motors.

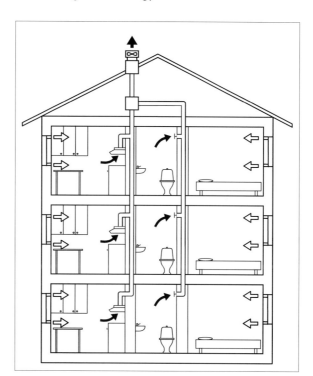

Figure 5. Mechanical exhaust ventilation system serving one or several apartments

In decentralized systems, more components require maintenance and are more widely spread out, but ventilation is easier to control by demand.

3.5.3 Hybrid (mixed-mode) ventilation

It is often possible to improve the reliability of natural ventilation or to increase the range over which low-energy ventilation methods can be applied by introducing mechanical assistance. Often, hybrid ventilation consists of no more than an auxiliary low-energy extract fan located in a natural ventilation extract duct. The fan is operated when driving forces are low or when priming a natural ventilation stack to prevent reverse flow. At the opposite extreme, a hybrid system can include a natural ventilation system combined with a fully independent mechanical system. In this case, natural ventilation is used for as long as climate and operational conditions permit, after which the mechanical system takes over. Efficiency can be improved by zoning the building so that some parts operate under natural conditions while others are mechanically ventilated. Depending on the approach, hybrid systems extend the applicability of ventilation to a wider range of buildings, including multi-storey buildings, urban locations and shopping malls.

Hybrid ventilation approaches may provide advantages in energy and cost over fully air-conditioned mechanical approaches in a wide variety of climatic regions and even in very complex buildings (Aggerholm, 2003).

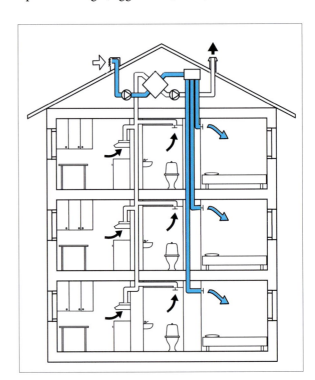

Figure 6. Centralized mechanical supply and exhaust system with heat recovery in an apartment building

3.6 Outdoor and other sources of pollution related to ventilation

Outdoor air used for ventilation may also be a source of pollution, containing particulate matter, particulates of biological origin (e.g. microorganisms and pollen) and various gases (e.g. nitric oxides and ozone). In naturally ventilated buildings, all pollutants in outdoor air enter the building. In mechanically ventilated buildings, it is possible to reduce the concentrations of pollutants in outdoor air before ventilation air enters. Nevertheless, the ventilation system may also be a source of indoor air contaminants.

3.6.1 Outdoor sources

Outdoor air intakes should be placed so that the air taken into a building is as clean as possible and, in summer, as cool as possible. Also, the air should not be polluted by sources close to the building. Potential outdoor sources of pollutants include: motor vehicle exhaust on busy streets, loading decks or garbage collection points; evaporative cooling systems and cooling towers (risk of *Legionella*); exhaust air openings and biomass-burning stoves and boilers. The arrangement of air intakes and discharge openings should also minimize the possibility of external recirculation between polluted exhaust air and clean air for ventilation.

Building envelopes and air cleaning appear to provide some protection from outdoor air pollutants (Hänninen at al., 2004). It has been suggested that ventilation systems in buildings could protect people from outdoor particles and their health effects (Fisk et al., 2002; Janssen et al., 2002; Leech, Raizenne, Gusdorf, 2004).

As people in high-income countries spend most of their time indoors, filtration of ambient pollution by building envelopes can be expected to be an important exposure modifier. In residential buildings, where mechanical ventilation systems have been rare, outdoor particles penetrate indoors very efficiently (penetration factors close to unity) (Özkaynak et al., 1996; Wallace, 1996), but, in buildings with two-way mechanical ventilation, air supply filters have been identified as the most significant means of particle removal (Thornburg et al., 2001). Hänninen et al. (2005) showed a 27% reduction in exposure to particulate matter measuring ≤ 2.5 μm in post- as compared with pre-1990 buildings due to mechanical ventilation with commonly used fine filters, which would correspond to eliminating all traffic exhaust particles in Helsinki. The use of air-conditioning systems was also suggested to contribute to a reduction in exposure to ozone and related health effects (Weschler, 2006).

3.6.2 Pollutants in air-handling equipment and systems

Several studies have shown that the prevalence of symptoms of sick-building syndrome is often higher in air-conditioned buildings than in buildings with natural ventilation (Mendell, Smith, 1990; Seppänen, Fisk, 2002). One explanation for the association between sick-building syndrome and mechanical heating, ventilating and air-conditioning systems is microbial and chemical pollutants, which are emitted by heating, ventilating and air-conditioning components and ductworks. Microbial growth on wet surfaces in air-handling systems can be a major source of pollution in old buildings. Mendell et al. (2007) corroborated their earlier findings (Mendell et al., 2006) that moisture-related heating, ventilation and air-conditioning components such as cooling coils and humidification systems, when poorly maintained, can be sources of microbiological contaminants that cause adverse health effects in occupants, even if the causal exposures cannot be identified or measured. Poor condition and maintenance of such systems in general has been identified as a risk factor (Mendell et al., 2003, 2006).

It has been also shown that sensory observations of chemical emissions from ventilation systems and heating and air-conditioning components are significant and play a major role in the perceived indoor air quality of a space (Fanger, 1988). The measured emission rates of volatile organic compounds from materials vary considerably (Morrison, Hodgson, 1996; Morrison et al., 1998). Materials with large emissions of volatile organic compounds are used in duct liners, neoprene gaskets, duct connectors and duct sealants, whereas high-surface-area materials, such as sheet metal, have lower emission rates. The emission of volatile organic compounds may increase when components and surfaces become dirty due to poor maintenance. This hypothesis is supported by the results of several field studies, which showed an association between indoor air problems and the dirtiness of heating, ventilation and air-conditioning systems (Sieber et al., 1996; Mendell et al., 2003). Siber et al. (1996) reported that an increased risk of multiple respiratory symptoms was related significantly to poor cleanliness of such systems (with a risk ratio (RR) of 1.8, to dirty filters (RR = 1.9), to debris in the air intake (RR = 3.1) and to dirty ductwork (RR = 2.1). All are indicators of sources of chemical pollutants in heating, ventilation and air-conditioning systems. Another major source of pollution is used air filters loaded with dust, which can react with other chemicals in the outdoor air and generate new chemicals that pass into the ventilation air through the filter (Wargocki, Wyon, Fanger, 2004).

The importance of clean air-handling systems has been recognized in national guidelines and standards in many countries (Verein Deutscher Ingenieure, 1997; Finnish Society of Indoor Air Quality and Climate, 2001; REHVA, 2007a,b; Pasanen, 2007).

Specific criteria for ventilation systems with regard to hygiene and other important factors are given in Box 3. More information is given in European Standard EN 13779 (CEN, 2007a) and ASHRAE standards 62.1 and 62.2 (ASHRAE, 2007a,b).

3.7 Ventilation and spread of contaminants

3.7.1 Ventilation and pressure differences in buildings

Ventilation, the stack effect and wind affect pressure differences over building structures. Pressure difference is a driving force for the airflows that transport water vapour and gaseous or particulate contaminants. One of the most important issues in respect of healthy buildings is keeping structures dry and preventing condensation of water in and on them. Convection of air and moisture through the building envelope can impose severe moisture loads on structures. In cold climates, the water content of the air is usually higher indoors than out.

BOX 3   **Specific criteria for ventilation systems**

Ventilation air should be distributed and used effectively in the building.
- Ventilation air should be distributed to the rooms of the building according to their design and use.
- In practice, therefore, the system should be designed and constructed so that airflow can be measured and balanced.
- Ventilation air should reach the breathing zone of the rooms as soon as possible after entering the room.
- Ventilation air should remove pollutants from the room effectively.
- Minimum ventilation rates should be increased when pollution loads are higher and can be lowered when pollution load is low.

Air used for ventilation should be clean.
- Outdoor air used for ventilation should not contain harmful chemicals, particles or odours (as in European Standard EN 13779).
- Air-handling systems should not degrade the quality of the air supply.

Ventilation air should not cause harm.
- It should not cause unacceptable thermal discomfort due to its temperature, velocity or flow direction.
- It should not cause acoustic discomfort, adverse health effects or difficulties in oral communication, but it can be used to mask more disturbing or annoying sounds, such as telephone conversations in open office spaces. (An example of criteria for noise levels is given in European Standard EN 15251.)
- It should not cause damage to building structures or operation. A ventilation system may create pressure differences in building structures that may lead to unwanted draughts close to doorways, difficulty in operating doors and moisture transport to the structures. (For an example of limit values for pressure differences, see European Standard EN 13779.)
- It should not spread pollutants from structures, the ground, outdoor air or indoor sources. Ventilation should enhance the air in a building by making it flow from clean areas to less clean areas. Ventilation should remove pollutants from their source (local exhaust). Pressure differences created by ventilation should not significantly increase the entry of polluted soil or air (radon and other harmful gases) into the building. Ventilation should not draw pollution from outdoor sources into the building (location of outdoor air intake). (Descriptive guidelines to avoid these problems are given in European Standard EN 13779.)

BOX 3 continues ▶

If the pressure is higher indoors, air with a high moisture content will flow into the cold structure, and water vapour may condense. The opposite is true in hot climates. Thus, exfiltration in cold climates and infiltration in hot climates can cause moisture accumulation or condensation, leading to microbial growth on materials, reduction of thermal insulation properties, changes in other material properties and even structural deterioration. The relative humidity at the junction of floors and external walls in multi-storey platform timber-frame houses can be high, resulting in a risk of mould growth and rot fungi when there is posi-

---

▶ BOX 3 continued

Ventilation should be provided to a building in an energy-efficient way.
■ Air for ventilation should be moved in an energy-efficient way. Natural forces should be used as much as possible. The use of electricity for fans should be limited. A value of 2.5 kW per m³/s (including supply and exhaust air fans) is used in Scandinavian guidelines. Heat recovery from ventilation air should be encouraged. The energy density in exhaust airflow is high, and heat recovery is often an economical way of reducing the energy and operation costs of ventilation. Heat recovery becomes more feasible with high air flows and low outdoor temperatures. Limit values can be set for minimum efficiency of heat recovery and the size of the air-handling system when heat is to be recovered.

Ventilation should be controllable by the occupants.
■ Individual control of ventilation should be encouraged, as it improves user satisfaction. Thus, individual control should be provided, if possible. Operable windows are one way to control ventilation and should be provided, particularly if the climatic conditions and location of the building are favourable for natural ventilation.

Quality control in design and construction
■ The design of ventilation requires professional skills. Criteria can be set for the person responsible for the design, as in Finland or the United States (professional engineers), where a building inspector checks the professional skills, training and experience of the principal designer.
■ One criteria for the proper design of ventilation is documentation, which is needed during the construction and operation of a building. The requirement for documentation may include design calculations, drawings and technical specifications.
■ Installation of ventilation requires professional skills. Criteria can be set for the person responsible for the installation, as in Finland, where a building inspector checks the professional skills, training and experience of the person in charge of the installation.
■ Tests, measurements and inspections by building inspectors and others may improve the quality of an installation. Guidelines for commissioning have been drawn up by engineering associations in Europe (Federation of European Heating and Airconditioning Associations) and in the United States (American Society of Heating Refrigerating and Air Conditioning Engineers).

Maintenance of ventilation systems
■ All ventilation systems require regular inspection and maintenance. An example of requirements is given in VDI 6022 (Verein Deutscher Ingenieure, 1997). Checklists for the hygienic operation and maintenance of air-conditioning systems are given in its appendix 3.1.

tive air pressure inside the building (Kilpeläinen et al., 2000). The simulation results of Janssens and Hens (2003) showed that, even when a roof design complies with condensation control standards, a lightweight system remains sensitive to condensation because of air leakage through the discontinuities, joints and perforations that are common to most construction methods.

The risk of condensation in buildings in cold climates can be reduced by higher exhaust flow rates than supply flow rates. In severe climates, especially, a pressure slightly lower indoors than outdoors (by not more than 20 Pa) can help avoid damage to structures caused by moisture. In hot, humid climates, the problem is reversed, and the supply airflow should be greater than the exhaust airflow. In a cold climate, buoyancy will cause a significant stack effect in winter. If the temperature difference is 40 °C, the pressure gradient in the room is about 2 Pa/m. In a two-storey house, this will lead to a positive pressure of 5 Pa on the first floor at ceiling height and –5 Pa at ground floor level when the air leakage

Figure 7. Pressure differences across a building envelope at 40 °C (red) and 20°C (blue) temperature difference between indoor and outdoor air

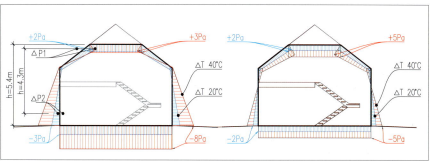

Source: Kurnitski *(2006).* In: Rakentajain kalentari, Rakennustieto Oy, 2006.
Note. The left-hand side of the figure shows measured results, including the effect of a ventilation system with a slightly higher exhaust than supply airflow rate. The right-hand side of the figure shows the calculated pressure differences caused by the stack effect only

flow paths are equally distributed. Figure 7 shows the measured and calculated results for a typical Finnish house with an average building leakage rate of four air changes per hour at a 50 Pa pressure difference; the air tightness of the building envelope is typically expressed by the airflow rate through the building envelope when the pressure difference between the outside and the inside is 50 Pa.

Field measurements and computer simulations of air pressure conditions in typical residences in a cold climate show that there is almost always a positive and a negative air pressure difference across the building envelope of detached houses and apartment buildings (Kalamees et al., 2007). In winter, continuous positive pressure is found at ceiling level on the top floor and negative pressure at floor level on the bottom floor. Wind influences air pressure peak values but not the average values. For detached houses, Kalamees et al. (2007) recommended a design value of ±10 Pa air pressure difference across the building envelope. They concluded that it is difficult to control air pressure differences in normal and leaky houses (air leakage rate, ≥ 4 air changes per hour at 50 Pa) with ventilation, as a $\pm$ 15% difference in airflow had only a minor influence on the air pressure difference. Pressure can be effectively controlled by ventilation only in extremely airtight houses (building leakage rate < 0.5 air changes per hour at 50 Pa).

Pressure differences are used in certain spaces (including buildings for human occupancy) designed for overpressure in relation to outdoor or adjacent spaces. Clean rooms, rooms for sensitive electronic data-processing equipment and operating theatres in hospitals are examples of such spaces. In buildings with no special requirements or emissions, ventilation systems are designed for neutral pressure conditions. Pressure conditions should be monitored continuously in spaces where there are heavy emissions of impurities. Also, the air pressures in stairways, corridors and other passages should be designed so that they do not cause airflow from one room or apartment to another.

3.7.2   Spread of gaseous and particulate contaminants, including mould products, by pressure differences

It has been suspected that airflow through mouldy structures carries harmful pollutants inside (Backman et al., 2000). Residential buildings often have mechanical exhaust ventilation, with intake air coming through inlets and cracks. In cold climates, inlets cause draughts in winter and are often closed, resulting in a high negative pressure indoors and forced airflow through cracks. Typically, mechanical exhaust ventilation creates a negative pressure of 5–10 Pa in apartments (Säteri, Kovanen, Pallari, 1999) if the inlets are open. A field study by Kurnitski (2000a) showed high infiltration airflow rates through leaks in a base floor to an apartment at a pressure difference of 6–15 Pa, which depended on the speed of the exhaust fan. Pessi et al. (2002) found that fungal spores can penetrate external sandwich wall structures when mechanical exhaust ventilation is used. Field measurements (Mattson, Carlson, Engh, 2002) showed that mould spores can be carried inside a house with mould growth in the crawl space through a base floor. The transport was highly dependent on exhaust ventilation, as the outdoor and indoor concentrations with non-operating ventilation were 200–500 CFU/ m^3, but when exhaust ventilation was switched on an indoor concentration of 5000 CFU/m^3 was measured. In field measurements in 10 residential buildings (Airaksinen et al., 2004b), the correlation between fungal spores in the crawl space and indoors depended on the microbial species. The concentration of the most abundant species, *Penicillium*, did not correlate with the indoor concentration, while that of *Acremonium* (which has no natural indoor source) did, indicating air leakage and fungal spore transport from crawl space air.

Crawl spaces and ground soil ventilated by outdoor air are typical locations for mould growth, and a significant amount of contaminated material can remain in structures even after repairs (Nguyen Thi, Kerr, Johanson, 2000). In contaminated crawl spaces, spore concentrations of 10^3–10^5 CFU/g of material samples are common (Kurnitski, Pasanen, 2000). The highest levels have usually been found on wood-based boards and timber. In cases of heavy fungal colonization, airborne spore concentrations of up to 10^3–10^4 CFU/m^3 have been detected. Kurnitski (2000b) and Airaksinen (2003) have shown that conditions are often favourable for microbial growth even in well-designed crawl spaces ventilated by outdoor air.

Many studies have been carried out to estimate the penetration of particles through cracks. Vette et al. (2001) report penetration factors (per number of particles) of 0.5–0.8 for particles of 0.5–2.5 µm. Mosley et al. (2001) found that, at a pressure of 5 Pa, 40% of 2-µm particles and less than 1% of 5-µm particles penetrated horizontal slits at a height of 0.5 mm. Liu and Nazaroff (2003) predicted that particles of 0.1–1.0 µm have the highest penetration efficiency, at nearly unity for crack heights of 0.25 mm or larger and a pressure difference of $\geq$ 4 Pa. These results are important, as the median aerodynamic diameter of fungi in indoor air is typically 2–3 µm (Macher, Huang, Flores, 1991; Reponen, 1995), which is suitable for penetration. About 70–90% of the viable fungi in indoor air are estimated to be in the respirable size fraction (Li, Kuo, 1994; DeKoster, Thorne, 1995).

Few studies have been carried out on particle penetration in the real structures commonly used in buildings. Liu and Nazaroff (2001) used a simulation model to predict that penetration through mineral wool insulation is negligible. In full-scale laboratory measurements, Airaksinen et al. (2004a) established that inert particles and fungal spores in the size range 0.6–2.5 mm penetrated a common wooden frame structure lined with mineral wool at moderate pressure differences of 6–20 Pa. Penetration was highly dependent on pressure differences and not on holes in the surface boards of the structure. It was proposed that the surface contact of mineral wool with other building elements plays an important role in penetration.

Relative pressure in a building, spaces and the ventilation system should be designed to prevent the spread of odours and impurities in annoying or harmful amounts or concentrations. The pressure conditions should not change significantly with changes in weather conditions. The airtightness of the building envelope, floors and partition walls, which affect the pressure conditions, should be defined at the design stage, by taking into account both temperature and wind conditions. The pressure relationships should be confirmed in the commissioning of a building and may be recommissioned periodically to ensure that deterioration of building components or shifting due to thermal, wind or seismic forces has not degraded the envelope tightness or other pressure-critical components.

3.8　Moisture control in buildings

Moisture control in buildings includes measures for choosing building materials and measures for controlling indoor humidity by ventilation (see section 3.4). In most climates (e.g. Europe), adequate ventilation, heating with adequate moisture control and thermal insulation of building structures will be enough to keep relative humidity on and in building structures within acceptable limits. Thus, microbial growth and dampness are usually indicators of construction faults, moisture damage, or malfunction of ventilation or heating systems.

Developments in building assemblies and materials and the requirements of good indoor climate and energy performance have resulted in wall, attic and floor assemblies that, once wet, take longer to dry and are more likely to allow condensation. Many contemporary assemblies contain materials that are more likely to support mould growth than the simple, often massive assemblies used in eras when the energy performance of a building was considered less important. When materials, methods and equipment change each year, it is no longer practical to wait for rules of thumb to emerge from generations of successful and failed buildings. Assemblies must be based on a better understanding of their thermal, moisture and airflow properties and those of their materials.

To control moisture, to ensure long building life and good indoor air quality, three goals must be set and met:

- control liquid water;
- manage indoor humidity levels and condensation; and
- select materials and hygrothermal assembly designs that minimize mould growth (see performance indicators in section 3.3) and other moisture problems.

For effective control of liquid water intrusion, measures must be applied during the design and construction phase, as well during operation and maintenance. Barriers to water entry should be established and maintained with capillary breaks in the building enclosure. Moisture migration by capillary action can be broken by an air space or water-impermeable material, such as drainage planes behind the cladding of wall assemblies. Precipitation shed from a building should be deflected by continuous, effective site drainage and a storm-water runoff system. Plumbing leaks can be prevented by locating plumbing lines and components where they are easy to inspect and repair, are unlikely to freeze and, if they leak, will not soak porous insulating materials. Building materials that are sensitive to moisture should be kept dry during transport and on-site storage; if they accidentally get wet, they should be dried before being enclosed into building assemblies.

Effective control of condensation requires careful design of building assemblies and heating, ventilation and air-conditioning systems. Continuous thermal barriers should be designed, installed and maintained to ensure that interior surfaces (including inside building assemblies) remain warm or cold, as designed. Building air pressure relationships should be controlled between indoor spaces and outdoors and between spaces to minimize the flow of warm, humid air towards cold surfaces. This affects and is affected by the design of both the enclosure and the heating, ventilation and air-conditioning system. Continuous air barriers should be designed and maintained to minimize infiltration of cold or hot, humid outside air into building assemblies or interior spaces. Also, heating, ventilation and air-conditioning systems should be designed, installed and maintained to manage indoor relative humidity and to effectively exhaust known sources of moist air.

Building assembly design should include selection of materials that minimize mould and other moisture problems – that is, building materials, equipment and design assemblies that can withstand repeated wetting in areas that are expected to get wet, such as spaces where water is used (kitchens and bathrooms) and below-grade wall and floor insulation and finishes.

Moisture control does not mean the elimination of water. Many materials can safely get wet, as long as they dry quickly enough. Others are so easily damaged by water that they must never get wet, like paper-faced gypsum board. Concrete, while porous and clean, is resistant to mould growth, contains no nutrients for mould or decay organisms and is stable when wet. It contributes to moisture problems only because it can wick liquid water to more vulnerable materials, and it takes a long time to dry.

Hygrothermal assembly design is an essential element for preventing moisture damage and guaranteeing longer service life for buildings. Several gaps in everyday design practice can affect potential moisture problems. Hygrothermal design consists of selecting and dimensioning structures, making detailed drawings and selecting specifications for critical joints and other documents and rules for operation and maintenance (Lehtinen, 2000). In many cases, hygrothermal design is conducted by engineers (architectural, structural and heating, ventilation and air-conditioning design) and has not been established as a separate area. To assess and predict the long-term hygrothermal performance of a building envelope, calculations or experimental investigations are needed. Because laboratory and field experiments are expensive and time-consuming, calculations and simulations are increasingly used to assess the hygrothermal behaviour of building components. During the past few decades, computer programs for simulation have been developed, and advanced commercially available simulation tools for personal computers have replaced laboratory tools; they are easy to use and include databases of building materials and climatic data (Kalamees, 2006).

According to Burke and Yverås (2004), the use of simulation tools in hygrothermal design by consulting companies is limited because they are too expensive, too difficult to learn and too time-consuming to run. This is perhaps the reason why, as a rule, hygrothermal dimensioning in consulting companies is limited to calculation of U-values and moisture accumulation in structures due to water vapour diffusion on the basis of the Glaser method (Lehtinen, 2000).

Nevertheless, consulting companies have had to use hygrothermal simulation programs in complicated renovation cases that require sophisticated analyses. In the design of new houses, the solutions already developed, tested and standardized are easier to use, accounting for the limited use of simulation tools.

In research, simulation tools are used to solve hygrothermal problems of building assemblies. There are good examples for crawl spaces (Kurnitski, 2000a; Airaksinen, 2003), attics and roofs (Salonvaara, Nieminen, 2002; Kalagasidis, Mattsson, 2005) and churches (Häupl, Fechnerm, 2003; Schellen et al., 2004). Such research leads to solutions for typical building envelopes in certain climatic areas (Burch, Saunders, 1995; Karagiozis, 2002; Mukhopadhyaya et al., 2003) and the hygrothermal performance of renovated building envelopes, such as internal thermal insulation (Cerny, Madera, Grunewald, 2001; Häupl, Jurk, Petzold, 2003). It is important that such results be taken into account in revision of building codes and guidelines.

3.9　Measures to protect against damage due to moisture

Moisture control is the main method for controlling mould and mites. The reasons for mould and mites are the same all over Europe, but the methods of control may differ. The effectiveness of a measure to control health determinants indoors can vary by climate, existing building construction, and heating, ventilation and air-conditioning systems.

Wet surfaces in air-conditioning and ventilation systems are always at risk of microbial contamination and pollution. Air-conditioning systems should be designed and operated so that microbial growth is avoided. Guidelines are available for hygienic design and operation of air-conditioning and ventilation systems (REHVA, 2007a,b), but the maintenance of air-handling systems is often neglected. It is important to keep all surfaces of an air-handling system clean.

The effectiveness of actions to control moisture also depends on whether they are for new or existing buildings. A wider variety of control methods can be applied in new constructions (Table 3) than in existing buildings (Table 4). Measures to control moisture may increase or decrease the construction or operation costs of a building, as indicated in the tables. In new constructions, most of the proposed measures reduce the operating costs by lowering energy consumption but slightly increase construction costs. It is particularly important to have an adequate ventilation rate in buildings when the thermal performance and airtightness are improved to meet energy performance criteria.

The measures against moisture damage described in Table 3 are grouped into three categories. The first group covers building construction. Structures should be designed, constructed and maintained so as to withstand the indoor humidity without harmful condensation of water vapour that migrates to the structure.

The second group covers ventilation. Its effect is twofold: it can remove indoor generated moisture directly and reduce the level of moisture. In some climatic

Table 3. Methods for controlling moisture in new buildings with better building codes

Method	Effect on construction cost	Effect on energy consumption and cost
Building construction		
Improve thermal properties of windows.	Increase	Decrease
Design structures to resist the moisture loads of local climate and typical use of buildings (e.g. use vapour barriers).	Negligible	None or small decrease
Ventilate walls and other building components to prevent condensation.	Negligible	None or small decrease
Improve thermal insulation of building envelope to increase indoor surface temperatures to prevent condensation in cold and moderate climates.	Increase	Decrease
Prevent moisture migration from ground by draining surface waters.	Negligible	None or small decrease
Improve protection by roofing, walls and windows against rain.	Negligible	None or small decrease
Design and install material for minimum leakage of plumbing.	Negligible	None
Ventilation		
Provide openable windows in all living rooms and kitchen.	Slight increase	May increase or decrease
Provide adequate, controllable average ventilation.	Slight increase	May increase or decrease
Ventilate all rooms where needed.	Slight increase	May increase or decrease
Provide effective kitchen range hood.	Slight increase	May increase or decrease
Provide possibility for controlling ventilation on demand.	Slight increase	Decrease
Use mechanical exhaust ventilation in warm and moderate climates; tighten building envelope to prevent excess ventilation.	Slight increase	Decrease due to reduced air leakage
Use mechanical supply and exhaust ventilation with heat recovery to reduce relative humidity indoors.	Slight increase	Decrease
Heating		
Use central heating in cold and moderate climates.	Slight increase	Slight increase
Do not use unvented open-flame heaters.	None	None
Control indoor temperature with thermostats.	Slight increase	Decrease
Encourage use of district heating.	Negligible	Decreases use of primary energy
Require chimneys for all heating boilers and furnaces.	Slight increase	Better efficiency; decrease in primary energy
Improve control of fireplaces with e.g. dampers or shutters; to improve the thermal efficiency of fireplaces.	Slight increase	Decrease

Source: Seppänen (2004)

Table 4. Methods for controlling moisture in existing buildings

Method	Effect on construction cost	Effect on energy consumption
Consumer behaviour and operation		
Limit use of humidifiers	None	Decrease
Do not dry laundry in living area	None	Decrease
Use kitchen range hoods and ventilation during cooking	None	Increase or decrease
Use ventilation and airing to prevent high indoor humidity and condensation	None	Increase or decrease
Increase indoor temperature to decrease relative humidity	None	Increase
Refurbishment		
Improve performance of ventilation (natural or mechanical)	Minor	Increase or decrease
Install mechanical ventilation system to improve ventilation (with or without heat recovery)	Medium	Decrease
Install double glazing to prevent condensation	Medium	Decrease
Improve roofing to prevent water leakages, when applicable	Medium	Decrease
Ventilate crawl spaces to prevent moisture migration from ground, when applicable	Small increase	None
Install range hoods in kitchen	Small increase	Increase or decrease
Replace unvented open-flame heaters and appliances with vented ones	Small increase	Improves efficiency and reduces primary energy use

Source: Seppänen *(2004).*

conditions (summer in some coastal areas), the outdoor moisture content may be high, and ventilation is not effective. The third group of measures covers heating. Effective central heating, preferably by cogenerated district heating, decreases indoor relative humidity and decreases the generation of moisture and pollutants from combustion.

In existing buildings (Table 4), the primary means for controlling moisture is changing consumer behaviour and improving ventilation. The measures for dealing with the building envelope are expensive and not as cost effective in the short term as those for ventilation. In the long term, however, ventilation measures may be more costly. Additional measures to reduce moisture can be taken by the occupants. Indoor relative humidity can depend on the air circulation in a room. Soft furniture, bookshelves close to exterior walls and carpets can increase the relative humidity indoors locally and cause mould growth. The relative humidity in carpets may be 10% higher than in room air; textile surfaces and carpets are good reservoirs for microbiological contamination and are very difficult to clean when contaminated. Heavy wall-to-wall carpeting is a risk factor in a humid climate.

Indoor air dehumidification can be used, in which dehumidified air is circulated through a cooling coil, where water is condensed and drained. After cooling and dehumidification, the air can be heated with the same device back to room temperature. These devices are particularly useful for temporary applications. From the standpoint of energy use, it is important that air be dehumidified to a relative humidity not much lower than the limit value for the growth of mites (45%).

The main methods for preventing moisture in buildings are summarized in Figure 8.

3.10 Conclusions and recommendations

While microbial growth and health outcomes are consequences, their common denominator is undesired moisture behaviour (i.e. excess moisture in building assemblies or on surfaces). The reasons for the presence of mould and mites are the same all over the world, but the methods of control may differ. Water intrusion, dampness and moisture-related phenomena are not only harmful for

Figure 8. Controlling moisture through building design and construction

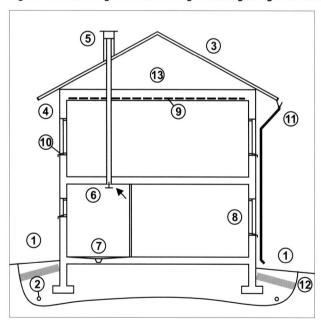

(1) Drain rainwater and surface water from near the building. (2) Drain the foundations with an underground pipe. (3) Install a tilted (rather than a flat) roof in wet climates. (4) Install eaves to protect walls from rain. (5) Install watertight piping penetrating the roof. (6) Install good ventilation, especially in bathrooms, laundry rooms and kitches. (7) Install watertight, sloping floors with floor drains in wet-process rooms. (8) Prevent condensation on walls and windows. (9) Install vapour barriers in walls. (10) Use good, watertight window construction, including window sills. (11) Drain rainwater from the roof. (12) Protect against frost when applicable. (13) Ventilate attics and crawl spaces when applicable.

occupants' health but are also a serious risk to building structures. In addition to risks of rotting wooden structures and microbial growth, building materials can also be degraded by chemical processes induced by moisture.

Moisture control, including ventilation, is the main method for containing mould and mites. The problems of building moisture and dampness, microbial contamination, repair and control practices vary by climate zone. Regardless of the climate, however, the prevention and control of moisture and the subsequent effects should be addressed in the early phases of building construction and by sustained maintenance.

Effective moisture control includes control of liquid water, control of indoor humidity levels and condensation and selection of materials and hygrothermal assembly design that minimize mould growth and other moisture problems. Dynamic simulations of heat and moisture and mould growth models are useful for assessing the hygrothermal performance of building assemblies. Methods should be further developed to allow calculation of fungal spore transport through building assemblies.

It is evident that a sufficient flow of outdoor air for ventilation is necessary: to remove indoor-generated pollutants and moisture from indoor air or to dilute their concentrations to acceptable levels for occupants' health and comfort; and to maintain building integrity. Ventilation can be provided by either natural or mechanical means, but both need careful implementation to avoid malfunctioning. Failures in ventilation may lead to serious health problems and damage to building construction.

4. Health effects associated with dampness and mould

Mark J. Mendell, Anna G. Mirer, Kerry Cheung, Jeroen Douwes, Torben Sigsgaard, Jakob Bønløkke, Harald W. Meyer, Maija-Riitta Hirvonen and Marjut Roponen

This chapter contains separate reviews and a synthesis of the epidemiological, clinical and toxicological evidence on the health effects of dampness and mould.

4.1 Review of epidemiological evidence

This section summarizes the epidemiological literature on the health effects of dampness and mould and other dampness-related agents, combining the conclusions of large previous reviews with newly reviewed findings for selected health outcomes.

4.1.1 Background

Epidemiological studies provide evidence to link dampness and dampness-related exposures to human health effects; however, in interpreting these studies, consideration must be given to their inherent strengths and weaknesses. Errors such as studying only samples instead of entire populations and bias related to sampling, measurement and confounding can distort risk estimates. In addition, the evidence from a body of studies may be distorted by publication bias, which reflects a tendency not to publish or to publish more slowly negative or equivocal findings, which may therefore not be included in the review.

In interpreting epidemiological studies on dampness, the uncertainty about the causal exposures and health effects involved must also be taken into account. Microbiological organisms are considered among the most plausible explanations for the health risks associated with indoor dampness. Conventional quantitative measurements of such exposure, however, based on counts of total culturable airborne microorganisms, have shown less consistent associations with the health effects of interest than have more qualitative assessments, such as visible dampness or water damage, visible mould or mould odour. While the association between qualitative assessments of dampness and health effects does suggest preventive strategies, the demonstration of specific, quantifiable causes would allow more effective prevention.

This review combines the conclusions of a review by the Institute of Medicine (2004), covering the literature up to mid-2003, those of a quantitative meta-analysis of findings up to 2007 on dampness, mould and respiratory health effects (Fisk, Lei-Gomez, Mendell, 2007) and a new assessment of more recent published studies on selected outcomes. The review focuses on selected categories of the outcomes included in the Institute of Medicine review (upper respiratory tract symptoms, cough, wheeze, dyspnoea, asthma symptoms in people with asthma, asthma development) and several additional categories (current asthma, respiratory infections, bronchitis, wheeze, allergic rhinitis and allergy or atopy). It excludes outcomes on which limited research has been reported (e.g. effects related to skin, eyes, fatigue, nausea, headache, insomnia, mucous membrane irritation and sick-building syndrome).

4.1.2 Methods

The online database PubMed was searched up to July 2007 for published articles, by using three groups of keywords, such as: (1) dampness, damp, water damage, moisture, humidity, fungi, fungus, mould, bacteria or microorganisms; along with (2) health, asthma, allergy, eczema, wheeze, cough, respiratory, respiratory infection, lung, skin, nasal, nose, hypersensitivity pneumonitis, alveolitis, bronchial, hypersensitivity or inflammation; and with (3) building, house, home, residence, dwelling, office, school or day-care centre. Some combinations of terms were searched separately. References in review articles or in personal databases were also included. Other references were added, as available.

For inclusion in this review, a study had to meet the following criteria:

- publication in a peer-reviewed journal (printed or online);
- reporting of original data from a study that was either an experimental intervention, a prospective cohort, a retrospective cohort or case-control, a cross-sectional or a cross-sectional case-control study;
- no minimum study size, except that if exposure was characterized only at building level, at least 10 buildings had to be included;
- it included risk factors related to dampness, fungi or microbiological components or products, other than allergens – such as those related to dust mites, cockroaches and mice;
- it included upper respiratory tract symptoms, cough, wheeze, dyspnoea, impaired lung function, allergy or atopy, asthma symptoms in people with asthma, asthma development, any diagnosis of asthma, current asthma, hypersensitivity pneumonitis, respiratory infections or bronchitis; and
- it provided adequate control, through the study design or analytical strategies, of selection bias and confounding by key variables: sex, active smoking (in studies of adults), passive smoking (in studies of children) and socioeconomic status (except in the Nordic countries).

Exposures and conditions that were not included were dust mites, humidity and measurements of moisture in mattresses. Endotoxins are components of Gram-negative bacteria that may favour moist surface conditions, but they are also associated with agricultural settings and with pets. A full consideration of the health effects of endotoxins was not included, as they are beyond the scope of this review, although findings of indoor endotoxin concentrations in studies of damp indoor conditions were included.

From each study, a limited set of data was abstracted, including the age of the participants, study design and point estimates and confidence intervals for specific combinations of risk factors or exposures. Studies were categorized as either interventions (controlled quasi-experimental field intervention studies), prospective (prospective cohort studies), retrospective (retrospective cohort or case–control studies) or cross-sectional (cross-sectional or cross-sectional case–control studies). The findings were organized into separate tables for each health outcome, and, within each table, the findings were sorted by the age of the participants and the study design.

The findings considered in evaluating the evidence were those of associations between health effects and qualitative assessments of dampness-related factors, such as visible dampness, mould, water damage or mould odour. Analyses based on quantified microbial exposures were considered secondary, as no specific microbial metric has been shown to be a consistent risk factor for health, and the evidence that a particular outcome is associated with a specific microbial measure is poor. Microbial metrics include culture-based assays of specific or total counts of fungi and bacteria, glucans, endotoxins, ergosterol and extracellular polysaccharides.

In this review, the quality of the evidence for a relation is classified in the same way as in the review of the Institute of Medicine (2004), as shown in Box 4. For each association considered, we classified the evidence on the basis of our professional judgement about the persuasiveness of the reported findings and consideration of the strength, quality, diversity and number of studies. The strongest epidemiological evidence was considered to be that from individually randomized controlled trials in which risk factors were added or removed, followed by prospective cohort and case–control studies, retrospective cohort and case–control studies and cross–sectional studies. A set of strongly designed studies of different designs and in different populations, with findings that were generally consistent in direction and magnitude, were considered to provide the most persuasive overall evidence, especially if they were bolstered by evidence from controlled studies of exposed human beings and experimental animals that demonstrated appropriate biological mechanisms for the epidemiological findings.

4.1.3 Results

4.1.3.1. Previous reviews

The most comprehensive, relevant reviews on dampness and health are those of Bornehag et al. (2001, 2004), the Institute of Medicine (2004) and Fisk, Lei-Gomez and Mendell (2007). Other reviews, opinion pieces and position statement on this topic were also available – for example, those of Peat, Dickerson and Li (1998), Kolstad et al. (2002), Hardin, Kelman, Saxon (2003), Douwes (2005), Hope and Simon (2007) and Mudarri and Fisk (2007).

A Nordic multidisciplinary committee (Bornehag et al., 2001) reported the findings of a review of the literature on dampness in buildings (including exposure to mites) and health, with conclusions based on 61 publications up to July 1998 that met the inclusion criteria. The review concluded that: "...dampness in buildings appears to increase the risk for health effects in the airways, such as

| BOX 4 | Classifying the strength of evidence |

The categories in this box refer to the association between exposure to an agent and a health outcome and not to the likelihood that any individual's health problem is associated with or caused by the exposure. These categories are used for classifying the evidence in this review and that of the Institute of Medicine (2004:26–27).

Sufficient evidence of a causal relationhip
The evidence is sufficient to conclude that a causal relationship exists between the agent and the outcome; that is, the evidence fulfils the criteria for "sufficient evidence of an association" and, in addition, satisfies the following evaluation criteria: strength of association, biological gradient, consistency of association, biological plausibility and coherence and temporally correct association.
The finding of sufficient evidence of a causal relationship between an exposure and a health outcome does not mean that the exposure inevitably leads to that outcome. Rather, it means that the exposure can cause the outcome, at least in some people under some circumstances.

Sufficient evidence of an association
The evidence is sufficient to conclude that there is an association. That is, an association between the agent and the outcome has been observed in studies in which chance, bias and confounding could be ruled out with reasonable confidence. For example, if several small studies that are free from bias and confounding show an association that is consistent in magnitude and direction, there may be sufficient evidence of an association.

Limited or suggestive evidence of an association
The evidence is suggestive of an association between the agent and the outcome but is limited because chance, bias and confounding could not be ruled out with confidence. For example, at least one high-quality study shows a positive association, but the results of other studies are inconsistent.

Inadequate or insufficient evidence to determine whether an association exists
The available studies are of insufficient quality, consistency or statistical power to permit a conclusion regarding the presence or absence of an association. Alternatively, no studies of the association exist.

Limited or suggestive evidence of no association
Several adequate studies are consistent in not showing an association between the agent and the outcome. A conclusion of no association is inevitably limited to the conditions, magnitude of exposure and length of observation covered by the studies available.

cough, wheeze and asthma… [and] evidence for a causal association between 'dampness' and health effects is strong. However, the mechanisms are unknown. Several definitions of dampness have been used in the studies, but all seem to be associated with health problems. Sensitization to mites may be one but obviously not the only mechanism. Even if the mechanisms are unknown, there is sufficient evidence to take preventive measures against dampness in buildings."

Three years later, the review was updated by a European multidisciplinary committee with 40 additional publications from 1998 through 2003 (Bornehag et al., 2004). This review concluded, "Dampness in buildings is a risk factor for health effects among atopics and nonatopics both in domestic and public environments. However, the literature is not conclusive in respect of causative agents…" Thus, the second review, somewhat more cautiously, did not claim that causality had been demonstrated in the literature reviewed.

The review of the Institute of Medicine (2004) was a detailed consideration of evidence available up to mid-2003 on the health effects of indoor dampness and dampness-related agents. The studies included in the review are summarized in Table A1.1 of Annex 1. This review, by an international multidisciplinary group, resulted in a book-length publication with an 87-page summary of the epidemiological evidence alone. The group drew conclusions about two categories of risk

Table 5. Findings of the review of the Institute of Medicine (2004)

Level of confidence for an association	Risk factor	
	Exposure to damp indoor environments	Presence of mould or other agents in damp indoor environments
Sufficient evidence of a causal association	No outcomes met this definition.	No outcomes met this definition.
Sufficient evidence of an association	Upper respiratory tract symptoms Wheeze Cough	Upper respiratory tract symptoms Wheeze Cough
	Asthma symptoms in sensitized people	Asthma symptoms in sensitized people Hypersensitivity pneumonitis
Limited or suggestive evidence of an association	Lower respiratory illness in otherwise healthy children Dyspnoea Asthma development	Lower respiratory illness in otherwise healthy children
Inadequate or insufficient evidence to determine whether an association exists	All other health effects considered	All other health effects considered

Reprinted with permission from "Damp, Indoor Spaces and Health" Washington, D.C, National Academies Press, 2004 factors: exposure to damp indoor environments and the presence of mould or other agents in damp indoor environments. Table 5 summarizes the conclusions of the review with regard to the epidemiological evidence on dampness-related health effects. Sufficient evidence was considered not to be available for any of the associations. Sufficient evidence of associations with exposure to damp indoor environments and with the presence of mould or other agents in damp indoor environments was considered to exist for four outcomes: upper respiratory (nose and throat) tract symptoms, cough, wheeze and asthma symptoms in sensitized people (i.e. asthma exacerbation). Sufficient evidence was also considered to exist for an association between dampness-related agents and hypersensitivity pneumonitis in susceptible persons. Table 6 shows the numbers of published studies included in the review, by study design for the health effect categories. It also shows the numbers of studies identified in the current review that were not included in the Institute of Medicine review. The results of the newly identified studies are discussed below.

Fisk, Lei-Gomez and Mendell (2007) reported the results of a quantitative meta-analysis on residential dampness-related risks for adverse respiratory health effects, which was based on studies available through early 2006 (which included most of the studies on specific outcomes used in the current review) and which met specified inclusion criteria. They estimated summary odds ratios and 95% confidence intervals for associations between dampness-related risk factors and six types of health outcome, including some of those in the Institute of Medicine review (upper respiratory tract symptoms, cough, wheeze and asthma development) and some other categories (current asthma and ever-diagnosed asthma). All types of visible dampness, mould or mould odour, reported by either occupants or researchers, were considered to represent a single set of dampness-related risks. Studies of measured concentrations of microbiological agents or of measured or reported air humidity were excluded. The results of the meta-analysis are summarized in Table 7. The central estimates of the odds ratio ranged from 1.34 to 1.75, with a lower confidence limit exceeding 1.0 in 9 of 10 estimates (i.e. for all except asthma development). The authors also estimated the percentage increase in prevalence of each outcome in houses with dampness or mould. Fisk, Lei-Gomez and Mendell (2007) concluded that "building dampness and mould are associated with approximately 30–50% increases in a variety of respiratory and asthma-related health outcomes." In a companion paper, Mudarri and Fisk (2007) estimated that, if the reported associations were causal, 21% of the cases of asthma in the United States could be attributable to dampness and mould in housing, for a total annual national cost of US$ 3.5 billion.

4.1.3.2. Additional published studies

The search conducted for the present review resulted in an initial 153 articles published between 1986 and 2007, excluding the 45 articles in the Institute of

Table 6. Numbers of published studies on health effects of damp indoor environments

Health outcome category	Included in review of the Institute of Medicine (2004)		Additional studies	
	Study design	No. of studies	Study design	No. of studies
Asthma development	Cohort	2	Prospective	3
	Case–control	6	Retrospective	2
	Cross-sectional	0	Cross-sectional	0
Current asthma	–	–	Prospective	1
			Retrospective	0
			Cross-sectional	17
Respiratory infections (in otherwise healthy people)	–	–	Prospective	3
			Retrospective	0
			Cross-sectional	5
Upper respiratory tract symptoms	Cohort	0	Prospective	1
	Case–control	0	Retrospective	0
	Cross-sectional	14	Cross-sectional	11
Allergic rhinitis	–		Prospective	3
			Retrospective	0
		–	Cross-sectional	3
Cough	Cohort	0	Prospective	1
	Case–control	1	Retrospective	0
	Cross-sectional	20	Cross-sectional	19
Wheeze	Cohort	0	Prospective	5
	Case-control	1	Retrospective	1
	Cross-sectional	19	Cross-sectional	24
Dyspnoea	Cohort	0	Prospective	0
	Case–control	0	Retrospective	0
	Cross-sectional	4	Cross-sectional	8
Altered lung function	–	–	Intervention	1
			Prospective	2
			Retrospective	0
			Cross-sectional	7
Bronchitis	–	–	Prospective	0
			Retrospective	0
			Cross-sectional	6
Other respiratory effects	–	–	Prospective	2
			Retrospective	0
			Cross-sectional	7
Allergy or atopy	–	–	Prospective	3
			Retrospective	0
			Cross-sectional	10
Asthma, ever	–	–	Prospective	2
			Retrospective	0
			Cross-sectional	6
Asthma symptoms in people with asthma	Intervention	0	Intervention	2
	Cohort	0	Prospective	1
	Case–control	5	Retrospective	0
	Cross-sectional	18	Cross-sectional	3
Total[1]		45		68

[1] Totals are less than the sum of the numbers above, as findings for several health effects may be reported.

Table 7. Key results of the meta-analyses of Fisk, Lei-Gomez and Mendell (2007)

Outcome	Participants	No. of studies	Odds ratio (95% CI)	Estimated % increase in outcome in houses with visible dampness, mould or mould odour
Upper respiratory tract symptoms	All	13	1.70 (1.44–2.00)	52
Cough	All	18	1.67 (1.49–1.86)	50
	Adults	6	1.52 (1.18–1.96)	–
	Children	12	1.75 (1.56–1.96)	–
Wheeze	All	22	1.50 (1.38–1.64)	44
	Adults	5	1.39 (1.04–1.85)	–
	Children	17	1.53 (1.39–1.68)	–
Current asthma	All	10	1.56 (1.30–1.86)	50
Ever-diagnosed asthma	All	8	1.37 (1.23–1.53)	33
Asthma development	All	4	1.34 (0.86–2.10)	30

Note. CI, confidence interval

Medicine review but potentially including articles in other reviews. Table 6 lists the 68 studies out of the 153 that met the inclusion criteria for this review (see section 4.1.2). Table A1.2 in Annex 1 summarizes the results of these studies by category of health outcome.

After an expert assessment of all the available evidence, including the studies analysed previously by the Institute of Medicine (Table A1.1) and the new studies found for this review (Table A1.2), we summarized the level of confidence for associations between dampness or dampness-related agents and specific health outcomes (Table 8).

The overall evidence shows that house dampness is consistently associated with a wide range of respiratory health effects, most notably asthma, wheeze, cough, respiratory infections and upper respiratory tract symptoms. These associations have been observed in many studies conducted in many geographical regions (Brunekreef et al., 1989; Jaakkola, Jaakkola, Ruotsalainen, 1993; Andriessen, Brunekreef, Roemer, 1998; Nafstad et al., 1998; Peat, Dickerson, Li, 1998; Norbäck et al., 1999; Øie et al., 1999; Bornehag et al., 2001; Kilpeläinen et al., 2001; Zheng et al., 2002; Zock et al., 2002; Jaakkola, Hwang, Jaakkola, 2005). Positive associations have been found in infants (Nafstad et al., 1998; Øie et al., 1999), children (Brunekreef et al., 1989; Andriessen, Brunekreef, Roemer, 1998; Zheng et al., 2002) and adults (Norbäck et al., 1999; Kilpeläinen et al., 2001; Zock et al., 2002), and some evidence was found for dose–response relations (Engvall, Norrby, Norbäck, 2001; Pekkanen et al., 2007). The evidence for associations with measured exposures to fungi or other microorganisms or microbial agents is less consistent, probably due to uncertainties in exposure assessment (see Chapter 2). For one health outcome, asthma exacerbation, we consider the evidence to be sufficient to document an association and almost sufficient to document causal-

Table 8. Level of confidence for associations between indoor dampness-related agents and health outcomes considered in this review

Updated conclusion	Outcome (in italics if conclusion changed)	Conclusion of the Institute of Medicine (2004)	Additional evidence from new data
Sufficient evidence of a causal relationship	None	None	
Sufficient evidence of an association	Asthma exacerbation	Sufficient evidence	More studies; close to sufficient evidence of causation
	Upper respiratory tract symptoms	Sufficient evidence	Many new studies, but not of improved quality
	Cough	Sufficient evidence	Many new studies, but not of improved quality
	Wheeze	Sufficient evidence	Many new studies, some of improved quality
	Asthma development	*Limited or suggestive evidence of association*	More studies of improved quality
	Dyspnoea	*Limited or suggestive evidence of association*	More studies
	Current asthma	*Not evaluated*	First evaluation
	Respiratory infections	*Not evaluated*	First evaluation
Limited or suggestive evidence of association	*Bronchitis*	*Not evaluated*	First evaluation
	Allergic rhinitis	*Not evaluated separately*	First evaluation
Inadequate or insufficient evidence to determine whether an association exists	Altered lung function	Not evaluated	First evaluation
	Allergy or atopy	Not evaluated	First evaluation
	Asthma, ever	Not evaluated	First evaluation

ity of dampness-related factors. A number of newly available studies added to the evidence of an association between dampness and asthma exacerbation. In all the available studies (Tables A1.1 and A1.2), dampness-related factors were consistently associated with asthma exacerbation, with odds ratios (ORs) consistently exceeding 1.0. This was true for both adults (in all case-control studies the ORs were 1.7–3.3, and in all cross-sectional studies the ORs were 1.02–4.2) and children (in all intervention studies; in all prospective studies the ORs were 3.8–7.6; in all case-control studies the ORs were 1.5–4.9; and in 96% of findings in cross-sectional studies the ORs were 1.0–7.6). Kercsmar et al. (2006) conducted a well designed, controlled intervention study on asthma exacerbation in the houses of highly symptomatic children with asthma and found that comprehensive removal of sources of dampness and mould and cleaning of visible mould dramatically reduced asthma exacerbation. This study (although of necessity unblinded) strongly suggests a causal association between indoor dampness or mould and respiratory morbidity in children with asthma.

We found that there was sufficient evidence for associations between indoor dampness and four health outcomes that were not so classified or were not evaluated by the Institute of Medicine (2004): asthma development, dyspnoea, current asthma and respiratory infections. Asthma development is a health outcome of particular public health importance. Five case–control studies included in the Institute of Medicine review (of the eight on asthma development in Table A1.1) explicitly addressed associations between dampness or mould and asthma development (Nafstad et al., 1998; Øie et al., 1999; Yang et al., 1998; Thorn, Brisman, Toren, 2001; Jaakkola et al., 2002). Four new studies were identified for the current review (Jaakkola, Hwang, Jaakkola, 2005; Matheson et al., 2005; Gunnbjornsdottir et al., 2006; Pekkanen et al., 2007), all of which were prospective or retrospective and reported effect measures exceeding 1.0 for most evaluations of dampness-related factors (see Table A1.2). Of the retrospective case–control studies of adults, 60% had ORs exceeding 1.0 (range, 0.8–2.2), and 74% of prospective or retrospective case-control studies in children had ORs exceeding 1.0 (range, 0.63–4.12). In both studies of infants, all the ORs exceeded 1.0 (range, 2.4–3.8); however, as asthma cannot be reliably assessed in infants, these findings should be interpreted with caution (Nafstad et al., 1998; Øie et al., 1999). These studies were not included in the meta-analysis of Fisk, Lei-Gomez and Mendell (2007), which found a summary OR of 1.3 (95% CI, 0.9–2.1) for asthma development and dampness factors.

The one study in which quantitative microbial measurements were used, a prospective study in adults, did not find consistent increases in risk (only 25% of ORs exceeded 1.0, ranging from 0.9 to 1.5). One of the strongest reported studies (Pekkanen et al., 2007), a retrospective case–control study of incident asthma cases, which was not included in the meta-analysis of Fisk, Lei-Gomez and Mendell (2007), showed that dampness or mould in the main living area of a house was related in a dose–response fashion to asthma development in infants and children. The multivariate-adjusted ORs for asthma incidence associated with three levels of maximum severity of moisture damage (assessed by civil engineers) were 1.0, 2.8 (95% CI, 1.4–5.4) and 4.0 (95% CI, 1.6–10.2). This well-designed study is the strongest available piece of evidence within a body of generally consistent findings that dampness-related exposure is not only associated with, but may cause, asthma in infants and children.

For dyspnoea, for which the Institute of Medicine considered there was limited or suggestive evidence of an association with dampness, the number of studies in adults and children had doubled to eight, although they were all still cross-sectional. In the available studies (Tables A1.1 and A1.2), the measures of association between dampness-related factors and dyspnoea were predominantly (81%) greater than 1.0, ranging from 0.41 to 9.38.

Current asthma, which was not evaluated in the Institute of Medicine review, was consistently associated in the available studies (Table A1.2) with qualitative markers of indoor dampness. In three cross-sectional studies of adults and 12 of children, almost all (91%) the ORs exceeded 1.0 (range, 0.36–12.99). Of the assessments with quantitative measurements of microbial exposure, the one prospective study of adults found predominantly (75%) elevated ORs for current asthma (range, 0.92–1.54), and three cross-sectional studies of adults or children also found mainly (81%) elevated ORs (range, 0.46–8.50). In their quantitative summary of effect estimates, Fisk, Lei-Gomez and Mendell (2007) reported an OR of 1.6 (95% CI, 1.3–1.9) for current asthma and dampness factors.

Respiratory infections were also not evaluated in the Institute of Medicine review. Of the available studies of qualitative dampness-related factors and respiratory infections (Table A1.2), besides the few results for otitis media, two prospective studies of children found consistently elevated ORs, ranging from 1.34 to 5.10, and five cross-sectional studies in children found mostly (73%) elevated ORs, ranging from 0.65 to 1.85. In studies with quantitative measurements of mould levels, two prospective studies of children had mixed findings, with 67% of ORs above 1.0 but ranging from 0.46 to 6.88. The few findings on otitis media, in three studies of children, showed estimates ranging from 1.0 to 1.37 for qualitative dampness factors and 0.72 to 3.45 for quantitative mould levels.

Outcomes evaluated in this review (Table A1.2) but not in that of the Institute of Medicine include allergic rhinitis, altered lung function, bronchitis, allergy or atopy and "asthma, ever". Completely consistent associations (100%) were found for bronchitis, but the evidence was limited to five cross-sectional studies. There was some suggestion that indoor dampness was associated with allergic rhinitis, but the evidence was inconsistent. The evidence for altered lung function, allergy or atopy and "asthma, ever" was considered insufficient due to the small number of studies, inconsistencies in the data or a combination of the two.

Our review did not include studies on the health effects of moisture and microbiological growth within heating, ventilation and air-conditioning systems, although these are potentially common effects in buildings with air-conditioning systems or humidification. A number of studies suggested increased risks of building-related symptoms, including lower respiratory tract symptoms, due to poorly designed or maintained heating, ventilating and air-conditioning systems (e.g. Sieber et al., 1996; Mendell et al., 2003, 2006) or simply due to the presence of air-conditioning systems, which produce moisture on cool surfaces of the systems, over which all the ventilation air to building occupants flows (Mendell, Smith, 1990; Mendell et al., 1996; Seppänen, Fisk, 2002; Bernstein et al., 2006). These effects appeared probably to be due to uncharacterized microbiological agents. The strongest study on this question is that of Menzies et al. (2003), which is a blinded, controlled, multiple cross-over intervention study in office buildings with no known contamination of heating, ventilation or air-conditioning systems or building-related health problems. The study showed that ultraviolet germicidal irradiation of the wet surfaces of cooling coils and condensate drip-pans in heating, ventilation and air-conditioning systems substantially reduced symptoms among the occupants. The findings suggest that microorganisms growing on moist surfaces in typical commercial air-conditioning systems can substantially increase building-related symptoms. The findings also imply that atopic people and nonsmokers are more responsive to microbiological agents in the form of increased respiratory and musculoskeletal symptoms. Thus, ultraviolet germicidal irradiation reduced the frequency of lower respiratory tract symptoms by 30% among current smokers but by 60% among people who had never smoked. This pattern of susceptibility is similar to that for hypersensitivity pneumonitis and may indicate a milder subclinical process. Hypersensitivity pneumonitis-like illness caused by indoor work environments has been reported repeatedly, generally in relation to leaks, but is considered rare (Kreiss, 1989). A possible explanation for these findings can be found in the reports of Gorny and others, who have shown that fungi and actinomycetes can emit large numbers of airborne particles smaller than spores (Gorny et al., 2002) (see Chapter 2).

4.1.3.3. Uncertainty

It is helpful to explore, as far as is feasible, how the findings of studies are influenced by various aspects of quality, including the quality of measurements of exposures and health outcomes. For instance, two reviews addressed the possibility that biased responses by building occupants in studies of dampness distort the findings. Fisk, Lei-Gomez and Mendell (2007) considered information on this question in six studies and concluded that the associations observed between respiratory health effects and dampness-related exposure were unlikely to be explained by overreporting of dampness or mould by people with respiratory symptoms. Bornehag et al. (2001) reported that the findings of studies with independent assessments of dampness and of health effects were similar to those of studies with more subjective sources of information.

The findings could also be compared on the basis of whether assessment of exposure was qualitative or quantitative. Random error in crude qualitative exposure categories tends to reduce the ability of studies to reveal true associations. The objective measures of exposure used in the studies have important limitations (see also Chapter 2). First, measurement of concentrations of culturable microorganisms is known to incur substantial error, due, for example, to short-term estimation of airborne concentrations that vary widely and rapidly over time, to the differential ability of organisms to grow on specific culture media and to the inability of culture assays to identify most bioactive microbial materials, whether intact spores or fragments. Second, the quantitative microbial measurements used in some of the studies cannot be considered to be inherently more accurate for assessing exposure, as the microbes may not be relevant causal factors. The exposures that cause dampness-related illness have not yet been determined. A study of an association between health effects and the concentration of a specific microorganism or microbial compound is in fact testing a hypothesis. In the studies in our review, such hypothetical causal exposures included all culturable fungi, specific culturable fungi, all fungal spores, species-specific spores, all fungal biomass (ergosterol) (Robine et al., 2005), the total mass of specific organisms (*Aspergillus* and *Penicillium* extracellular polysaccharides) and specific toxic compounds (endotoxins, β-glucans).

Avoidance behaviour is another source of exposure misclassification; that is, people with asthma might change their living environment to reduce exposure. This is a concern mainly in cross-sectional and case-control studies, in which it can lead to an underestimate of the true effect. It is of no concern in those studies in which exposure is assessed before the onset of asthma.

Finally, the lack of standardization of the definitions of health effects can result in bias. In population studies, for instance, asthma is usually defined on the basis of self-reported (or parent-reported) asthma symptoms, which include wheeze, chest tightness, breathlessness and cough. Self-reports of doctor-diagnosed asthma are also often used. An alternative to questionnaires has been the use of more objective measures, such as bronchial responsiveness testing, either alone or in combination with questionnaires. As with measures of house dampness or fungal exposure, differences in asthma definition are likely to result in different estimates of prevalence and of relative risks. Also, as mentioned above, several studies (Nafstad et al., 1998; Øie et al., 1999) evaluated infants, in whom a diagnosis of asthma is less certain than in older children. Most of these potential sources of bias can result in underestimates of the true association between indoor damp and health effects.

4.1.4   The hygiene hypothesis

Many studies have found that health risks are increased by exposure to microbes, but others suggest that exposure in early life to endotoxins or fungal agents protects against atopy and allergic disease. This potentially protective effect is consistent with the hygiene hypothesis, which postulates that growing up in a microbiologically hygienic environment might increase the risk of developing allergies (Liu, Leung, 2006). This hypothesis was prompted by the results of epidemiological studies showing that overcrowding and unhygienic conditions were associated with lower prevalences of allergies, eczema and hay fever (Strachan, 1989). A more recent review confirmed the associations between large family size, low socioeconomic status and hepatitis A infection and decreased risks of atopy, hay fever or eczema, but not for asthma (Strachan, 2000). Exposure to certain microbial agents, including bacterial endotoxins, early in life has been proposed as an explanation for these protective effects (Douwes et al., 2004). Several cross-sectional studies showed significant inverse associations between indoor endotoxin levels and atopic sensitization, hay fever and atopic asthma (Gereda et al., 2000; Gehring et al., 2002; Braun-Fahrländer, 2003).

A recent prospective birth cohort study showed an inverse association between the levels of both bacterial endotoxins and fungal components measured at three months on the floor and doctor-diagnosed asthma and persistent wheeze at age 4 years, confirming some of the earlier findings of the cross-sectional studies (Douwes et al., 2006). A similar birth cohort study found a protective effect against atopy in children aged 2 years (Bottcher et al., 2003); however, this was not confirmed in another birth cohort study, which showed that early exposure to endotoxins was associated with an increased risk of atopy at the age of 2 years (Bolte et al., 2003). Several studies have shown reduced risks of atopy, hay fever, asthma and eczema among farmers' children and adolescents; although the specific protective factors were not identified, the authors suggested that endotoxins and other microbial agents play an important role (Douwes, Pearce, Heederik, 2002; Douwes et al., 2004).

The evidence has not, however, been consistent (Liu, 2007; von Mutius, 2007). Several large studies showed either no protective effect or even a positive association. For instance, the National Survey of Allergens and Endotoxin in Housing in the United States showed an exposure-dependent increase in diagnosed asthma, wheeze and use of asthma medication in adults with increasing endotoxin concentrations in the bedroom floor and bedding (Thorne et al., 2005). Michel et al. (1996) showed that endotoxins in floor dust and high exposure to dust mites were positively associated with the severity of asthma in people who were also allergic to house dust mites,. Some of the inconsistency may be due to the timing of exposure, being protective in early life and being a risk factor later in life. Alternatively, exposure to endotoxins may prevent allergic asthma, but at higher exposure may cause non-allergic asthma (Douwes, Pearce, Heederik, 2002).

It is provocative that many well-conducted studies showed apparent protective effects of measured exposures to microbial agents, such as endotoxins and fungi. Douwes et al. (2006) reported the results of a prospective study that showed strongly protective associations between both endotoxins and extracellular markers of *Penicillium* or *Aspergillus* and doctor-diagnosed asthma. Other studies have shown that greater exposure to endotoxins is associated with decreased risks of atopy (Gehring et al., 2002; Bottcher et al., 2003) and asthma (Braun-Fahrländer et al., 2002). Li and Hsu (1997) reported the results of a cross-sectional study in which the concentrations of culturable *Penicillium* in indoor air were inversely associated with allergic rhinitis. Iossifova et al. (2007) reported that a prospective study showed that β-glucan was protective against recurrent wheezing in infants. The findings are not, however, consistent. For instance,

Dharmage et al. (2001) found that exposure to high indoor air levels of *Cladosporium* and *Penicillium* decreased the risk of fungal sensitization, but they found that these fungi were associated with high risks of bronchial hyperresponsiveness. Osborne et al. (2006) found that increased exposure of infants to *Cladosporium* was associated with a reduced risk of atopy, although exposure to *Penicillium*, *Aspergillus* and *Alternaria* was associated with an increased risk.

Braun-Fahrländer (2003) cautioned that "exposure to endotoxin might partly be a surrogate measure of a much broader spectrum of immunomodulatory microbial compounds." If in fact exposure to certain microbiological agents early in life protects against atopy and asthma, it is puzzling that no similar pattern is seen for dampness-related risk factors in infants. Overall, the available evidence is still inconsistent, and further research is required for clarification.

Thus, modest exposure to microbial agents may, under certain circumstances, protect against allergies and allergic disease, but the evidence is inconsistent. There is no indication that living or working in a damp building with heavy exposure to mould prevents the development of allergies and respiratory disease.

4.1.5 Conclusions

Our review of the epidemiological evidence presented in this report, the previous review by the Institute of Medicine and the quantitative meta-analysis of Fisk, Lei-Gomez and Mendell (2007) leads us to conclude that there is sufficient evidence of an association between indoor dampness-related factors and a wide range of respiratory health effects (Table 8), including asthma development, asthma exacerbation, current asthma, respiratory infections, upper respiratory tract symptoms, cough, wheeze and dyspnoea. As we did not perform a formal meta-analysis, we cannot make a quantitative assessment of the relative risk; however, the quantitative summary estimates of associations between qualitatively assessed dampness or mould in residences and selected respiratory health effects provided by Fisk, Lei-Gomez and Mendell (2007) (Table 7) are valid, as few additional studies of this type have become available. Their estimates suggest that a substantial increase in a number of important respiratory health outcomes, including a 50% increase in current asthma, is associated with dampness-related risk factors in residences. In an associated paper, it was estimated that, if these associations are causal, 21% of the cases of asthma in the United States could be attributed to residential dampness and mould (Mudarri, Fisk, 2007). As these estimates are based on limited data, broad lumping of diverse risk factors and multiple unverified assumptions, they should be interpreted cautiously; however, they do indicate that dampness-related risk factors may contribute substantially to the burden of respiratory disease.

Indoor dampness also appears to be associated with bronchitis and allergic rhinitis, but the evidence is either mixed (allergic rhinitis) or based on relatively few studies (bronchitis). For all the other health effects considered (altered lung function, allergy or atopy and "asthma, ever"), we consider the evidence to be inadequate or insufficient to determine whether an association exists.

In agreement with the Institute of Medicine (2004), we consider that there is insufficient evidence of a causal relationship with any of the health outcomes reviewed, although for asthma exacerbation we consider that there is almost enough evidence to meet the criteria of causality for dampness-related agents. The evidence does not suggest that any one measurement of microbiological materials is demonstrably more specific or sensitive for assessing dampness-related exposure that is relevant to health effects. Thus, although it is plausible that heavy exposure to indoor mould or other microbial agents plays a causal role, this has not been established conclusively.

4.1.4.1. Limitations of the approach

The restricted scope of this review resulted in a number of limitations. The method used to evaluate the evidence was largely non-quantitative; thus, all the available tools for summarizing the scientific literature could not be used. Furthermore, the conclusions of this review were derived primarily from findings based on qualitative measures of dampness-related factors. It is thus difficult to link the conclusions to specific exposures. It is also likely that publication bias influenced the results, inflating the association between risk factors and health effects. Formal application of statistical methods for assessing bias was beyond the scope of this review. We did not search for unpublished findings, which would have decreased publication bias. The conclusions drawn from this review should thus be considered provisional until a more thorough consideration of all the available findings is possible. It is recommended that the evidence for publication bias be addressed in a future review, with updated, quantitative summary estimates of risk.

4.2   Clinical aspects of health effects

This section focuses on studies involving human volunteers or experimental animals exposed in controlled circumstances, occupational groups or clinically. Most of these studies are based on small groups of individuals, but both the exposure and the clinical outcomes are characterized better than they are in the epidemiological studies.

4.2.1   β-glucans

Numerous studies have shown that β-glucans have important effects on the human immune system. β-glucan was identified as the biologically active component of immune-stimulating yeast cell extracts in 1961 (Riggi, Di Luzio, 1961). Since then, their effects, particularly in relation to infection and cancer, have been investigated extensively. The research has focused almost entirely on orally or intravenously administered glucans, however, and few studies have been conducted of experimental exposure of humans to mould or glucans; nevertheless, a series of studies was performed with healthy volunteers by Rylander and colleagues in Sweden.

In the first study, it was found that exposure to pure β-glucan (particulate curdlan at 210 ng/m³ for 4 hours) did not significantly affect lung function (Rylander, 1996), although some exposure-related irritation in the nose and throat occurred. A second experiment, with another β-glucan (grifolan in saline at about 30 ng/m³ for 3 hours), resulted only in an increased blood level of tumour necrosis factor alpha (TNF-α) (Beijer, Thorn, Rylander, 1998). In their third study, 125 ng of inhaled grifolan resulted in TNF-α, eosinophil cationic protein and neutrophils in sputum 24 hours later (Thorn, Brisman, Toren, 2001). These short-term exposures to pure glucan preparations cannot be compared directly with exposure to measured levels in buildings, which rarely exceed 100 ng/m³ of β-glucan. In a Danish study of 36 volunteers exposed to dust and glucan in a climate chamber, decreased nasal volume and increased interleukin (IL)-8 indicated that glucan enhanced the inflammatory effect of the dust on the upper airways (Bønløkke et al., 2006). In an unusual method of exposure, in which aqueous solutions of β-glucan (curdlan) were instilled directly into the nostrils of recycling workers, an increase in nasal volume was observed (Sigsgaard et al., 2000). In contrast, no volume changes were observed after instillation of a solution of *A. fumigatus* or compost.

Experimental inhalation by healthy non-allergic people of *A. fumigatus* allergen extract increased the amount of nitric oxide exhaled from their lungs and in nasal lavage fluid (Stark HJ et al., 2005; Stark et al., 2006). The authors also found indications of pro-inflammatory effects in nasal lavage fluid (increases in TNF-α and IL-1β), although the latter effect was obscured by an insufficient interval between exposure to the placebo and the mould. In another study in Denmark, with double-blind, placebo-controlled exposure of people who had previously experienced building-related symptoms after exposure to spores from two different moulds, no clinical effects were observed (Meyer et al., 2005). An intriguing lack of increase in blood neutrophils on the days of exposure to mould, as compared with the normal diurnal increase after placebo, might have been due to neutrophil extravasation elsewhere in the body. 3-methylfuran, a common fungal volatile compound, was found to increase blinking frequency and enzymes from neutrophilic granulocytes and to affect lung function at a concentration of 1 mg/m³, without causing symptoms (Walinder et al., 2005). This concentration is substantially higher than those measured in buildings.

Unfortunately, all the studies performed so far have been small and had insufficient statistical power to detect weak clinical effects. Exposure was to different components or preparations of mould, and, although concentrations were reported, none of the studies obtained sufficient information to calculate dose. In summary, mediators of inflammation and signs of inflammatory reactions tend to appear, with little change in symptoms, after exposure to a variety of low toxicity mould components; the effects appeared to be greater after 24 hours than immediately after exposure. Although some of the studies included people who were atopic or otherwise considered susceptible, the studies provide too limited evidence to allow conclusions about differences in susceptibility among healthy people. A number of studies have been performed in which guinea-pigs were exposed to β-glucans by inhalation. β-glucans that are insoluble in water appeared not to elicit a significant inflammatory response on inhalation; however, when a water-soluble β-glucan, such as schizophyllan, was used or an insoluble β-glucan was rendered soluble by treatment with sodium hydroxide, more leukocytes appeared in bronchoalveolar lavage fluid (Fogelmark et al., 1992). Grifolan treated with sodium hydroxide was found to cause airway eosinophilia (Fogelmark, Thorn, Rylander, 2001). Milanowski (1998) reported significant acute increases in neutrophilic granulocytes (polymorphonuclear leukocytes), lymphocytes and erythrocytes in bronchoalveolar lavage fluid after inhalation of β-(1,3)-glucan from Baker yeast suspended in saline. Several β-glucans, including insoluble forms, have been shown to modulate the response to other agents, such as endotoxins (Fogelmark et al., 1992; Fogelmark, Sjöstrand, Rylander, 1994; Fogelmark, Thorn, Rylander, 2001), cigarette smoke (Sjöstrand, Rylander, 1997) and ovalbumin (Rylander, Holt, 1998; Wan et al., 1999). Concomitant exposure to endotoxins and curdlan, a (1-3)-β-glucan, was shown to diminish the acute neutrophil response but to augment chronic inflammatory effects (Fogelmark, Sjöstrand, Rylander, 1994; Rylander, Fogelmark, 1994). Thus, the effects of inhalation of β-glucans apparently depend on the type of glucan as well as on concomitant exposures.

Several studies have linked β-glucan-contaminated environments to symptoms and signs of airway inflammation. Increased airway responsiveness to methacholine (Rylander, 1997b), amplified peak flow variation in children (Douwes et al., 2000) and a higher prevalence of atopy (Thorn, Rylander, 1998) have been associated with long-term occupation of buildings with high concentrations of airborne β-glucan. In these buildings, symptoms such as dry cough (Rylander et al., 1989, 1992, 1998a), nasal and throat irritation (Rylander et al., 1989), hoarseness (Rylander et al., 1998a) and tiredness and headache (Rylander et al., 1989; Wan et al., 1999) were found to be more prevalent. A few cases have also been published in which inhabitants of houses with signs of mould and with airborne glucan levels > 100 ng/m³ were severely afflicted with asthma-like symptoms until they moved (Rylander, 1994; Rylander et al., 1998a). These studies linking glucan with symptoms and signs of disease are insufficient to conclude that there is a causal relationship with glucan, which may be just a marker of exposure to another agent.

Waste handlers were found to have a work-related increase in polymorphonuclear leukocytes in nasal lavage fluid, which is related to biomarkers of inflammation, in particular to IL-8. The inflammatory response and swelling of the nasal mucosa were associated with exposure to glucan and fungal spores (Heldal et al., 2003). In another study, greater lymphocytosis was found at higher β-glucan levels (Thorn et al., 1998). In other occupations, no significant associations have been found between airway inflammation and exposure to β-glucans, although β-glucan levels are elevated during farming (Eduard et al., 2001; Roy, Thorne, 2003).

4.2.2 Mycotoxins

Mycotoxins are secondary metabolites produced by fungi, which can cause a toxic response in animals and human beings, often at very low concentrations. Many studies in vitro and in experimental animals have demonstrated the toxic potential of a variety of mycotoxins, including trichothecenes and sterigmatocystin (Institute of Medicine, 2004; Rocha, Ansari, Doohan, 2005).

It has been speculated that inhalation of aflatoxins and ochratoxin in industries such as peanut and livestock feed processing and industries in which exposure to grain dust occurs might increase the incidences of liver cancer, cancers of the biliary tract and salivary gland, and multiple myeloma (Olsen, Dragsted, Autrup, 1988; Selim, Juchems, Popendorf, 1998). A direct association with cancer has not been demonstrated, although adduct formation with aflatoxin has been found in such workers (Autrup et al., 1991). Inhaled mycotoxins have also been suggested to play a role in adverse reproductive outcomes among farmers (Kristensen, Andersen, Irgens, 2000).

Although mycotoxins can induce a wide range of adverse health effects in both animals and human beings, the evidence that they play a role in health problems related to indoor air is extremely weak. Nonetheless, one group of mycotoxins that has received considerable attention in this respect are the trichothecenes produced by S. chartarum. In a report from the Centers for Disease Control and Prevention (1994, 1997; Etzel et al., 1998), indoor exposure to these mycotoxins was suggested to be associated with acute pulmonary haemorrhage in a cluster of 10 infants presenting at the Cleveland Children's Hospital in 1993–1994. Pulmonary haemorrhage is characterized by strongly elevated levels of haemosiderin, an iron-containing pigment, in lung tissues. The condition can be fatal due to diffuse bleeding or haemorrhage in the alveoli. It is not commonly associated with bioaerosol exposure. These findings were later criticized by others on the basis of shortcomings in the collection, analysis and reporting of data and were retracted (Centers for Disease Control and Prevention, 2000), and the role of S. chartarum is still controversial. In view of these uncertainties, the Institute of Medicine (2004) concluded that "available case-report information, taken together, constitutes inadequate or insufficient information to determine whether an association exists between acute idiopathic pulmonary hemorrhage and the presence of S. chartarum." A subsequent study showed that people exposed to satratoxin in their houses form albumin adducts in their blood, as found in rats exposed experimentally to satratoxin G. This small study shows that exposure to high levels of *S. chartarum* in houses might have a biological effect (Yike et al., 2006).

4.2.3   Allergic alveolitis

Allergic alveolitis, also known as extrinsic allergic alveolitis and hypersensitivity pneumonitis, is an inflammatory disease involving the distal proportions of the airways. The disease has an immunological component, but it has been difficult to find the immunological mechanism by which antigens create granulomatous lymphocytic inflammation in the alveoli and bordering regions.

Allergic alveolitis is diagnosed with various clinical and paraclinical tests, including pathological examination and imaging of the lungs (for a comprehensive review, see Wild, Lopez, 2001). Although IgG antibodies were initially believed to be causative, they have been shown to be only markers of exposure (Marx et al., 1990; Cormier, Belanger, 1989; Malmberg et al., 1985). There have been sporadic case reports of allergic alveolitis in indoor environments in Europe and the United States (Torok, de Weck, Scherrer, 1981; Pedersen, Gravesen, 1983; Fergusson, Milne, Crompton, 1984; Bryant, Rogers, 1991; Siersted, Gravesen, 1993; Wright et al., 1999), often in connection with the use of humidifiers (von Assendelft et al., 1979; Nordenbo, Gravesen, 1979).

In Japan, more than 60 cases of allergic alveolitis caused by the mould *Trichosporon cutaneum* occur every year during the hot and humid summer season, with an incidence of 0.5 per 10^6 person–years (Ando et al., 1991, 1995). During this season, *T. cutaneum* grows rapidly, especially in wooden houses. It occurs only south of 40° latitude. A 10-year survey was conducted of all hospital cases of this condition throughout Japan, with diagnostic criteria including comprehensive paraclinical tests and confirmation of causality by a positive challenge test either to the environment or to the mould spores themselves. The survey showed that cases were concentrated in the southern part of Japan and occurred predominantly among housewives, who therefore spent most of their time in and around a building. Similar cases have been recently reported in the Republic of Korea and in southern Africa (Swingler, 1990; Yoo et al., 1997).

A smaller series in Finland consisted of seven cases of rhinitis and four of allergic asthma, one of which included allergic alveolitis, among 14 employees at a military hospital infested with *Sporobolomyces salmonicor* (Seuri et al., 2000). The cases of asthma and allergic alveolitis were confirmed by inhalation provocation with *S. salmonicor* from the hospital.

In case series of allergic alveolitis in the home environment and in industrial cases, the affected person is often in the same environment as the general population. Therefore, susceptibility must play a significant role. Familial clustering has been found (Allen, Basten, Woolcock, 1975), but the causative factor has not been identified (Schwarz, Wettengel, Kramer, 2000). It is striking that the vast majority of cases occur in nonsmokers.

The Institute of Medicine (2004) concluded that clinically significant allergic alveolitis occurred only in susceptible people exposed to sensitizing agents. The studies indicated that there is sufficient evidence of an association between the presence of mould and bacteria in damp indoor environments and allergic alveolitis. The only new study since that evaluation is that of Seuri et al. (2000), which does not change this conclusion.

4.2.4 Inhalation fever

Inhalation fever, also known as toxic pneumonitis, humidifier fever and organic dust toxic syndrome, is a self-limiting syndrome that occurs after inhalation of a wide range of substances, from metal fumes to bacteria and mould spores. The syndrome was first described as humidifier fever during the time when reservoir humidifiers were used. Outbreaks typically occurred during the heating season in museums, printing shops and other localities in which it was important to control the humidity in the environment (Rask-Andersen et al., 1994). Studies of farmers showed that the exposure to mould spores that leads to inhalation fever exceeds the levels that induce allergic alveolitis by one or two orders of magnitude (Rask-Andersen, 1988).

4.2.5 Infection with mould

Infection with *Aspergillus* and other fungi such as *Fusariuum* spp. is a well-known complication in the treatment of patients who are immune compromised due, for example, to treatment for cancer or infection with human immunodeficiency virus (Iwen et al., 1994, 1998; Geisler, Corey, 2002; Lednicky, Rayner, 2006). Some of these patients contract mould infection after exposure indoors, not because of water damage in the facilities where they are being treated but because an opportunistic, ubiquitous mould finds a suitable host. No studies have been conducted to link such infections to mould in the indoor environment. Furthermore, the type of disease appears to determine the type of infection, and the infecting agents are not those typically encountered in damp houses.

Aspergillus appears to be the most aggressive of these fungi, giving rise to infections also in patients with less severe airway disease, such as cystic fibrosis, asthma and chronic obstructive pulmonary disease. People who are atopic sometimes contract a severe infection in which aspergillosis causes an allergic reaction with the infection, giving the person wheeze, pulmonary infiltrates and eventually fibrosis (Kauffman, 2003). This syndrome can also be found with an aspergilloma (i.e. a tumour in a lung cavity consisting of *Aspergillus* hyphae) (Tanaka, 2004).

People with atopy sometimes develop sinus disease as a consequence of *Aspergillus* infection or presence (Dufour et al., 2006). Exposure to mould has been proposed as the cause of chronic sinusitis, as these patients show exaggerated humoral and cellular responses, both T(H)1 and T(H)2 types, to common airborne fungi, particularly *Alternaria* (Shin et al., 2004).

4.2.6   Other effects

Several other effects of exposure to mould have been discussed in the context of indoor air, including toxic, immunological, reproductive and neuropsychiatric symptoms and syndromes. The Institute of Medicine (2004) found no evidence that the prevalences of cancer and reproductive outcomes were altered by exposure to indoor air. A search of these subjects showed no studies on this subject within the past 5 years. The Institute of Medicine (2004) included only a few case reports, with inconsistent findings for neuropsychiatric effects.

A Finnish group studied the occurrence of rheumatic diseases associated with dampness. In two studies, the authors found clustering of cases of rheumatic disease in water-damaged buildings (Myllykangas-Luosujärvi et al., 2002; Luosujärvi et al., 2003) and suggested that the symptoms could be attributed to exposure to mould spores. In a later publication (Lange, 2004), the author proposed that endotoxins and other triggers of the innate immune response might play a role, although the exposure levels are much lower than those in situations where joint pain is more prevalent, as on farms and among bird fanciers. Rheumatic diseases among people exposed in damp buildings and the possible role of endotoxins was also reported by Lorenz et al. (2006).

4.3   Toxicological mechanisms

This brief review of toxicological studies on microbial exposure in damp buildings is based mainly on studies published between 2000 and mid-2007; when appropriate, references are also be made to earlier publications, including those in the review of the Institute of Medicine (2004). The data reviewed originate from studies in vitro (i.e. experimental studies in a controlled environment outside a living organism, such as a test tube), summarized in Table A2.1, and studies in experimental animals in vivo (Table A2.2). Although direct extrapolation from experimental data to human risk is not possible, the studies that are described provide important information about the possible toxicological mechanisms behind the observed health effects in damp buildings. This review focuses on the ability of microbial exposures associated with damp buildings to activate the following potential toxicological mechanisms: immunostimulation and allergies, cytotoxicity and immunosuppression, autoimmunity, irritation, neurotoxicity, genotoxity and reproductive toxicity. Novel toxicological data on the role of microbial interactions are also included.

The variety of respiratory symptoms and diseases observed in damp and mouldy indoor environments suggests that the airways are the primary route of entry for agents. Therefore, studies in experimental animals were limited to those in which the airways were used as the pathway of exposure, thus excluding the extensive literature on the induced toxic effects of bacterial toxins and mycotoxins, associated, for example, with ingestion of mould-contaminated food. Most of the in vitro and in vivo studies included in this review addressed the effects of microbial components found in damp buildings, such as fungal spores, bacterial spores and cells, and the toxic components or products of microbes (e.g. fungal mycotoxins and endotoxins) (see Tables A2.1 and A2.2). Possible toxic effects due to released non-microbial chemicals are not addressed, because experimental data on exposures to chemicals in damp buildings were missing or limited.

In damp buildings, people are exposed to constantly changing concentrations of different microbial species, their spores, metabolites and components, and other compounds in indoor air, including chemical emissions from building materials. This complex mixture of exposures inevitably leads to interactions, which may change the toxic characteristics of the inhaled particles, causing different outcomes in different situations. Furthermore, the effects of microorganisms, microbial substances or dampness-related chemical compounds seen in experimental animals or cells often result from exposures that are orders of magnitude higher than the average doses that reach the human lungs under normal conditions in indoor air. Nevertheless, the surface doses within the lungs of patients with respiratory conditions can vary a thousandfold, due to uneven particle deposition (Phalen et al., 2006), resulting in even larger maximal surface doses in human lungs than in those used in experimental toxicological studies. Moreover, many other factors, such as exercise, can result in larger-than-average doses in the human lung.

Thus, experimental toxicological studies are essential for clarifying cellular mechanisms and identifying causative compounds, but the dosage must be considered in interpreting the findings and attempting extrapolation to the range of human exposures indoors.

4.3.1   Immunostimulation and immunoglobulin E-mediated allergies

There is evidence that dampness in buildings increases the risks of asthma, sensitization and respiratory symptoms, as extensively reviewed by Bornehag et al. (2001, 2004). Many of the health effects may result from recurrent activation of immune defence, leading to exaggerated immune responses and prolonged production of inflammatory mediators. Overproduction of these compounds damages the surrounding tissues and may manifest itself as chronic inflammation and inflammation-related diseases, such as asthma (Martin, Frevert, 2005). The central role of inflammatory responses is corroborated by studies reporting increased levels of inflammatory mediators in nasal lavage fluid and induced sputum from the occupants of damp buildings (Hirvonen et al., 1999; Purokivi et al., 2001; Wålinder et al., 2001).

The immunostimulatory activity of Gram-negative bacterial lipopolysaccharide is well established, but several other bacteria, fungi and isolated mycotoxins associated with damp buildings have been shown to induce inflammatory responses in vitro (Huttunen et al., 2001; Nielsen et al., 2002; Huttunen et al., 2003; Pylkkänen et al., 2004; Johannessen, Nilsen, Lovik, 2005; see also Table A2.1). In line with the findings in vitro, the same microbial species activate acute (Nikulin et al., 1996; Rao, Brain, Burge, 2000; Jussila et al., 2003; Leino et al., 2003; Rand et al., 2006) and sustained inflammation in the lungs of experimental animals (Jussila et al., 2002a) (Table A2.2).

Furthermore, it has been shown in an animal model that immunological status plays an important role in airway inflammation induced by *S. chartarum*, enhancing the effects of the mould (Leino et al., 2006). The results imply that sensitized people are more susceptible to exposure to mould than nonatopic people. Different microbial species differ significantly in their immunostimulatory potency in both mouse and human cells in vitro (e.g. Huttunen et al., 2003). Furthermore, it has been clearly demonstrated that different growth conditions and competition between microorganisms for the same habitat in vitro change their inflammatory potency, protein expression and toxin production (Ehrlich, 1987; Meyer, Stahl, 2003; Murtoniemi et al., 2003).

One of the mechanisms underlying the health effects of exposure to microbial agents may be IgE-mediated allergic responses. Although many of the reported symptoms are similar to those of allergy, only a small percentage of exposed people actually develop allergies to mould (Taskinen et al., 1997; Immonen et al., 2001). The most prevalent fungal genera associated with mould allergy are *Aspergillus*, *Cladosporium* and *Penicillium* (Ledford, 1994). Sensitization to *A. alternata* has been linked to the development, persistence and severity of asthma (Zureik et al., 2002; Bush, Prochnau, 2004; Salo et al., 2006). Some fungal species can induce histamine release by other mechanisms (Larsen et al., 1996); thus, allergy-like symptoms can also occur in non-sensitized people. Some of the chemical compounds associated with damp and degrading materials, such as phthalates and their metabolites, can stimulate the immune system by acting as allergens or adjuvants (Hansen et al., 2007).

4.3.2 Cytotoxicity and immunosuppression

Increased frequencies of common respiratory infections have been observed in people living or working in damp buildings (Åberg et al., 1996; Pirhonen et al., 1996; Kilpeläinen et al., 2001), suggesting that agents present in the indoor air of these buildings can suppress immune responses, leading to increased susceptibility to infections. Several microbes originating from damp buildings or their toxins have been shown to have immunosuppressive effects in vitro mediated – for example, by impaired particle clearance (Pieckova, Jesenska, 1996, 1998) or by cytotoxicity (Huttunen et al., 2004; Penttinen et al., 2005a,b).

The immunosuppressive effects of mycotoxins have been confirmed in experimental animals. Trichothecenes T-2 and deoxynivalenol (vomitoxin) impair immune responses to respiratory virus infection, increasing the severity of infection (Li et al., 2006; Li M et al., 2007). Some airborne fungi and bacteria may act as opportunistic human pathogens, causing upper or lower airway, pulmonary and in some cases systemic infectious diseases in immunocompromised people (Bush et al., 2006).

The acute cytotoxicity of fungal strains in damp buildings has been found to be due to the metabolite profile produced in vitro, although their biological activity may not depend solely on toxin production (Nielsen et al., 2002; Huttunen et al., 2003). Fungal spores appear to have toxic effects other than those that cause the inflammatory reaction. Studies of Gram-positive and -negative bacteria (e.g. *Streptomyces californicus, Pseudomonas fluorescens, Mycobacterium terrae, Bacillus cereus*) have shown that the significant difference in cytoxicity among strains (Huttunen et al., 2003) is due at least partly to differences in inflammatory activity. Spores and toxins of the fungus *S. chartarum* have been shown to activate the apoptotic pathway (programmed cell death) (Islam et al., 2006; Wang, Yadav, 2006; Penttinen et al. 2007), whereas the spores of *S. californicus* induce cell cycle arrest (Penttinen et al., 2005b).

Studies in experimental animals with the same fungal or bacterial species confirm the in vitro findings for cytotoxic effects, showing increases in total protein and lactate dehydrogenase in bronchoalveolar lavage fluid from exposed animals, as well as lung tissue damage (Nikulin et al., 1996; Rao, Brain, Burge, 2000; Rao, Burge, Brain, 2000; Jussila et al., 2001, 2002a, 2002c; Yike et al., 2002; Jussila et al., 2003; Rand et al., 2006).

4.3.3 Autoimmunity

Cases of autoimmune diseases and related symptoms have been reported among the occupants of damp buildings (Myllykangas-Luosujärvi et al., 2002; Luosujärvi et al., 2003), but there are no toxicological data on autoimmune responses caused by microorganisms or microbial substances found in damp buildings. Microbial fragments can, however, cause autoimmune reactions by molecular mimicry, acting as microbial superantigens or by enhancing the presentation of autoantigens (Wucherpfennig, 2001).

4.3.4 Irritation

Spores and other particulate material, as well as volatile organic compounds produced by microorganisms, building materials, paints and solvents, are potentially irritating. In epidemiological studies, the prevalence of respiratory and irritative symptoms has been associated with perceived mould odour, possible indicating the presence of microbial volatile organic compounds (Jaakkola, Jaakkola, Ruotsalainen, 1993; Ruotsalainen, Jaakkola, Jaakkola, 1995). It has been suggested that these compounds are present in damp buildings at levels sufficient to cause symptoms of irritation in exposed people (Hope, Simon, 2007). Furthermore, the sensation of unpleasant odours as such can cause stress responses and nonspecific somatic symptoms such as headache and nausea.

4.3.5 Neurotoxicity

Such health effects as fatigue, headache and difficulties in concentration (Johanning et al., 1996; Koskinen et al., 1999b) indicate that microbes or other agents present in damp buildings have neurological effects.

Many pure microbial toxins, such as the products of *Fusarium* (fumonisin B1, deoxynivalenol), *Stachybotrys* (satratoxin G), *Aspergillus* (ochratoxin A) and *Penicillium* (ochratoxin A, verrucosidin), have been shown to be neurotoxic in vitro and in vivo (Rotter, Prelusky, Pestka, 1996; Belmadani et al., 1999; Kwon, Slikker, Davies, 2000; Islam, Harkema, Pestka, 2006; Stockmann-Juvala et al., 2006). No study has shown, however, that people living in damp buildings who complain of nervous system symptoms are exposed to effective levels of mycotoxins.

4.3.6 Genotoxicity

Heavy occupational exposure by inhalation to mycotoxins in mouldy grain may be linked to an increased risk of cancer (Olsen, Dragsted, Autrup, 1988; Kristensen, Andersen, Irgens, 2000), but there is no epidemiological evidence for an association between exposure in damp buildings and cancer. Some of the microbial toxins produced by bacteria and fungi are known to be genotoxic and carcinogenic (IARC, 1993), but the relevance of these findings to exposure by inhalation in damp buildings is not known. It has been shown, however, that microbial isolates from damp buildings have genotoxic activity in vitro. Wang and Yadav (2006) showed that toxins of *S. chartarum* extracted from spores cause DNA damage, *p53* accumulation and apoptosis in murine alveolar macrophages. Another report suggested that the spores of *S. californicus* produce genotoxically active compound(s) that induce DNA damage, and that the production of this compound is potentiated when the microbe grows together with *S. chartarum* (Penttinen et al., 2007). Microbial compounds may not only produce genotoxic compounds but may also increase the risk of cancer through secondary mechanisms (e.g. by inducing oxidative stress in chronic inflammation) (Fitzpatrick, 2001).

4.3.7 Reproductive toxicity

No studies were found on the effects of exposure to microbes in damp buildings on reproductive responses. One group of indoor air contaminants, phthalates, are, however, potential reproductive and developmental toxicants (Lottrup et al., 2006).

4.3.8 Microbial interactions

The immunostimulatory properties of the fungal and bacterial strains typically found in moisture-damaged buildings are synergistically potentiated by microbial interactions during concomitant exposure in vitro (Huttunen et al., 2004).

These interactions are not limited to microbes grown separately (Penttinen et al., 2005a) but also occur also when microbes are cultivated together (Penttinen et al., 2005b). Interactions between *S. californicus* and *S. chartarum* during co-cultivation stimulated the production of currently unidentified cytostatic compound(s) (Penttinen et al., 2006), which significantly potentiate the abilities of the spores to cause apoptotic cell death (Penttinen et al., 2005b). Interactions during co-cultivation stimulate these microbes to produce highly toxic compounds, which can damage DNA and provoke genotoxicity (Penttinen et al., 2007). In addition, concomitant exposure in vitro with amoebae potentiates the cytotoxic and inflammatory properties of the microbial spores of *S. californicus* or *Penicillium spinolosum* isolated from damp buildings (Yli-Pirilä et al., 2007). These findings point to the importance of considering microbial interactions when investigating the causative agents and mechanisms of the adverse health effects observed in damp buildings.

4.4 Synthesis of available evidence on health effects

In this chapter, we have presented several types of evidence – epidemiological, clinical and toxicological – relevant to answering the question of whether dampness or dampness-related exposures cause adverse human health effects. This summary is based initially on the epidemiological and clinical evidence for causal relations between dampness-related factors and specific human health outcomes. Then, the available toxicological evidence is considered as either supporting or not supporting the biological plausibility of any potentially causal association. The epidemiological evidence is based on qualitative assessments of dampness-related factors, such as visible dampness, mould, water damage or mould odour, as the epidemiological findings based on quantitative measurements of specific microbial agents were too inconsistent and, for specific outcomes, too few for clear conclusions.

The epidemiological evidence is not sufficient to conclude causal relationships between indoor dampness or mould and any specific human health effect, although the findings of one strong epidemiological intervention study, in conjunction with the other available studies, suggest that dampness or mould exacerbates asthma in children.

There is sufficient epidemiological evidence of associations between dampness or mould and asthma development, asthma exacerbation, current asthma, respiratory infections (except otitis media), upper respiratory tract symptoms, cough, wheeze and dyspnoea. There is sufficient clinical evidence of associations between mould and other dampness-associated microbiological agents and hypersensitivity pneumonitis, allergic alveolitis and mould infections in suscep-tible individuals, and humidifier fever and inhalation fevers. This is the only con-clusion that is based primarily on clinical evidence and also the only conclusion that refers explicitly to microbial agents, as opposed to dampness-related factors.

Limited or suggestive epidemiological evidence of an association between in-door dampness or mould and allergic rhinitis and bronchitis is available.

The evidence for effects on lung function, allergy or atopy and "asthma, ever" is inadequate or insufficient. The evidence does not suggest that any specific measure of microorganisms or microbial substances results in a demonstrably more specific or sensitive assessment of a particular dampness-related exposure relevant to health effects. Nonetheless, although specific causal agents have not been identified conclusively, microbial exposure is often suggested to play a role. Further studies with valid, quantitative exposure assessment methods are re-quired to elucidate the role of fungi and other microorganisms in damp-induced health conditions. The available epidemiological and clinical evidence suggests that both atopic and nonatopic people are susceptible to adverse health effects from exposure to dampness and mould, even if some outcomes are commoner in atopic people. Therefore, both allergic and non-allergic mechanisms may be involved in the biological response.

The mechanisms by which non-infectious microbial exposures contribute to adverse health effects associated with indoor air dampness and mould are largely unknown. It is clear, however, that no single mechanism can explain the wide variety of effects associated with dampness and mould. Toxicological studies, by investigating the ability of microbial agents associated with damp buildings to activate certain toxicological mechanisms, provide insight into the multiple biological mechanisms that might underlie the observed associations between health effects and dampness and mould. In vitro and in vivo studies have demon-strated diverse inflammatory, cytotoxic and immunosuppressive responses after exposure to the spores, metabolites and components of microbial species found in damp buildings, lending plausibility to the epidemiological findings.

Many dampness-associated conditions are likely to involve inflammation, as inflammatory responses to many microbiological agents have been found. These include histamine release by mechanisms other than those mediated by IgE, in-dicating a plausible mechanism for the occurrence of allergy-like symptoms even in non-sensitized people. Dampness-associated asthma, allergic sensitization and associated respiratory symptoms may result from repeated activation of the immune defences, exaggerated immune responses, prolonged production of in-flammatory mediators and tissue damage, leading to chronic inflammation and inflammation-related diseases, such as asthma.

Although fungal spores associated with damp buildings produce metabolites with demonstrated acute cytotoxicity, the spores also have toxic effects other than those caused by the inflammatory reaction. The observed increase in the frequency of respiratory infections associated with damp buildings might be explained by the immunosuppressive effects of damp building-associated microbes in experimental animals, which impair immune defences and thus increase susceptibility to infections. An alternative explanation might be that inflamed mucosal tissue provides a less effective barrier, increasing the risk of infection. Demonstration of such effects in cells or experimental animals at levels of microbial exposure similar to those in indoor environments would allow extrapolation of these results to human beings.

Various microbial agents with diverse, fluctuating inflammatory and toxic potential are present simultaneously with other airborne compounds, inevitably resulting in interactions in indoor air. Such interactions may lead to unexpected responses, even at low concentrations. Therefore, the detection of individual exposures, such as certain microbial species, toxins or chemical agents, cannot always explain any associated adverse health effects. In the search for causative constituents, toxicological studies should be combined with comprehensive microbiological and chemical analyses of indoor samples.

The synergistic interactions among microbial agents present in damp buildings suggest that the immunotoxic effects of the fungal and bacterial strains typically found can be potentiated during concomitant exposure, leading, for instance, to increased cell death or cytotoxic or inflammatory effects. Such interactions can give rise to unexpected responses, even at low concentrations of microbial (or chemical) agents, so that it is difficult to detect and implicate specific exposures in the causation of damp building-associated adverse health effects. Thus, microbial interactions must be carefully considered when evaluating the possible health effects of exposure in damp buildings. Differences in the concentrations used in studies with cell cultures or experimental animals and those that may be reached by human beings should also be kept in mind when interpreting the findings.

Most of the relevant toxicological data from studies in experimental animals refer to the immunotoxicity of fungi, especially the species *S. chartarum* and its toxins. The role of other microbial exposures, including dampness-related bacteria, requires more study. For the identification of causative constituents and risk assessment, toxicological and epidemiological data should be combined with microbiological and chemical analyses of indoor air samples. In interpreting the results of studies in experimental animals in relation to human exposures, it is important to consider differences in relative doses and the fact that the exposures used for experimental animals may be orders of magnitude higher than those found in indoor environments.

The available estimates, based on the assumption that the associations found in the epidemiological studies are unbiased and causal, suggest that dampness-related risk factors are associated with a large proportion of human respiratory disease. For instance, residential dampness is associated with a 50% increase in current asthma and substantial increases in other respiratory health outcomes, suggesting that 21% of current asthma in the United States may be attributable to residential dampness and mould (Fisk, Lei-Gomez, Mendell, 2007; Mudarri, Fisk, 2007). These estimates, for imprecisely defined risk factors, cannot indicate true causal relationships and must be interpreted with caution, but they suggest that some dampness-related risk factors contribute substantially to the burden of human respiratory disease.

5. Evaluation of human health risks and guidelines

5.1   Summary

Sufficient epidemiological evidence is available from studies conducted in different countries and under different climatic conditions to show that the occupants of damp or mouldy buildings, both houses and public buildings, are at increased risk of respiratory symptoms, respiratory infections and exacerbation of asthma. Some evidence suggests increased risks of allergic rhinitis and asthma. Although few intervention studies are available, their results show that remediation of dampness problems can reduce adverse health outcomes.

There is clinical evidence that exposure to mould and other dampness-related microbial agents increases the risks of rare conditions, such as hypersensitivity pneumonitis, allergic alveolitis, chronic rhinosinusitis and allergic fungal sinusitis. Toxicological evidence obtained in vivo and in vitro supports these findings, showing the occurrence of diverse inflammatory and toxic responses after exposure to microorganisms – including their spores, metabolites and components – isolated from damp buildings.

While groups such as atopic and allergic people are particularly susceptible to biological and chemical agents in damp indoor environments, adverse health effects have also been found in nonatopic populations.

The increasing prevalences of asthma and allergies in many countries increase the number of people susceptible to the effects of dampness and mould in buildings.

5.2   Conditions that contribute to health risks

The prevalence of indoor dampness varies widely within and among countries, continents and climate zones. It is estimated to affect 10–50% of indoor environments in Australia, Europe, India, Japan and North America. In certain settings, such as river valleys and coastal areas, the conditions of dampness are substantially more severe than the national average.

The amount of water available on or in materials is the most important trigger of the growth of microorganisms, including fungi, actinomycetes and other bacteria.

Microorganisms are ubiquitous. Microbes propagate rapidly wherever water is available. The dust and dirt normally present in most indoor spaces provide sufficient nutrients to support extensive microbial growth. While mould can grow on all materials, selection of appropriate materials can prevent dirt accumulation, moisture penetration and mould growth.

Microbial growth may result in greater numbers of spores, cell fragments, allergens, mycotoxins, endotoxins, β-glucans and volatile organic compounds in indoor air. The causative agents of the adverse health effects have not been identified conclusively, but an excess level of any of these agents in the indoor environment is a potential health hazard.

Microbial interactions and moisture-related physical and chemical emissions from building materials may also play a role in dampness-related health effects. Building standards and regulations for comfort and health do not sufficiently emphasize requirements for preventing and controlling excess moisture and dampness.

Apart from its entry during occasional events, such as water leaks, heavy rain and flooding, most moisture enters buildings in incoming air, including that infiltrating though the envelope, or from the occupants' activities. Allowing surfaces to become cooler than the surrounding air may result in unwanted condensation. Thermal bridges (such as metal window frames), inadequate insulation and unplanned air pathways, or cold water plumbing and cool parts of air-conditioning units can result in surface temperatures below the dew point of the air and in dampness.

5.3   Guidelines

Persistent dampness and microbial growth on interior surfaces and in building structures should be avoided or minimized, as they may lead to adverse health effects.

Indicators of dampness and microbial growth include the presence of condensation on surfaces or in structures, visible mould, perceived mould odour and a history of water damage, leakage or penetration. Thorough inspection and, if necessary, appropriate measurements can be used to confirm indoor moisture and microbial growth.

As the relationships between dampness, microbial exposure and health effects cannot be quantified precisely, no quantitative, health-based guideline values or thresholds can be recommended for acceptable levels of contamination by microorganisms. Instead, it is recommended that dampness and mould-related problems be prevented. When they occur, they should be remediated because they increase the risk of hazardous exposure to microbes and chemicals.

Well-designed, well-constructed, well-maintained building envelopes are critical to the prevention and control of excess moisture and microbial growth, as they prevent thermal bridges and the entry of liquid or vapour-phase water. Management of moisture requires proper control of temperature and ventilation to avoid excess humidity, condensation on surfaces and excess moisture in materials. Ventilation should be distributed effectively throughout spaces, and stagnant air zones should be avoided.

Building owners are responsible for providing a healthy workplace or living environment that is free of excess moisture and mould, by ensuring proper building construction and maintenance. The occupants are responsible for managing the use of water, heating, ventilation and appliances in a manner that does not lead to dampness and mould growth.

Local recommendations for different regions with different climates should be updated to control dampness-mediated microbial growth in buildings and to ensure desirable indoor air quality.

Dampness and mould may be particularly prevalent in poorly maintained housing for low-income people. Remediation of the conditions that lead to adverse exposure should be given priority to prevent an additional contribution to poor health in populations who are already living with an increased burden of disease.

6. References

Åberg N et al. (1996). Prevalence of allergic diseases in schoolchildren in relation to family history, upper respiratory infections, and residential characteristics. *Allergy*, 51:232–237.

Adan OCG (1994). *On the fungal defacement of interior finishes* [thesis]. Eindhoven, Eindhoven University of Technology.

Aggerholm S (2003). Control of hybrid ventilation systems. *International Journal of Ventilation*, 1:65–76.

Airaksinen M (2003). *Moisture and fungal spore transport in outdoor air ventilated crawl spaces in a cold climate* [thesis]. Espoo, Helsinki University of Technology, Department of Mechanical Engineering, Laboratory of Heating, Ventilating and Air Conditioning.

Airaksinen M et al. (2004a). Fungal spore transport through a building structure. *Indoor Air*, 14:92–104.

Airaksinen M et al. (2004b). Microbial contamination of indoor air due to leakages from crawl space: a field study. *Indoor Air*, 14:55–64.

Aketagawa J et al. (1993). Activation of *Limulus* coagulation factor G by several (1→3)-β-D-glucans: comparison of the potency of glucans with identical degree of polymerization but different conformations. *Journal of Biochemistry*, 113:683–686.

Al-Khatib I et al. (2003). Impact of housing conditions on the health of the people at al-Ama'ri refugee camp in the West Bank of Palestine. *International Journal of Environmental Health Research*, 13:315–326.

Allen DH, Basten A, Woolcock AJ (1975). Familial hypersensitivity pneumonitis. *American Journal of Medicine*, 59:505–514.

Alper Z et al. (2006). Risk factors for wheezing in primary school children in Bursa, Turkey. *American Journal of Rhinology*, 20:53–63.

Alvarez AJ et al. (1994). Use of solid-phase PCR for enhanced detection of airborne microorganisms. *Applied and Environmental Microbiology*, 60:374–376.

Andersson MA et al. (1998). The mitochondrial toxin produced by *Streptomyces griseus* strains isolated from an indoor environment is valinomycin. *Applied and Environmental Microbiology*, 64:4767–4773.

Ando M et al. (1991). Japanese summer-type hypersensitivity pneumonitis. Geographic distribution, home environment, and clinical characteristics of 621 cases. *American Review of Respiratory Diseases*, 144:765–769.

Ando M et al. (1995) Summer-type hypersensitivity pneumonitis. *Internal Medicine*, 34:707–712.

Andriessen JW, Brunekreef B, Roemer W (1998). Home dampness and respiratory health status in European children. *Clinical and Experimental Allergy*, 28:1191–1200.

Arlian LG (1992). Water balance and humidity requirements of house dust mites. *Experimental and Applied Acarology*, 16:15–35.

Arundel AV et al. (1986). Indirect health effects of relative humidity in indoor environments. *Environmental Health Perspectives*, 65:351–361.

ASHRAE (2007a). *ANSI/ASHRAE standard 62.1-2007: Ventilation for acceptable indoor air quality*. Atlanta, American Society of Heating Refrigerating and Air Conditioning Engineers.

ASHRAE (2007b). *ANSI/ASHRAE standard 62.2-2007: Ventilation and acceptable indoor air quality in low-rise residential buildings*. Atlanta, American Society of Heating Refrigerating and Air Conditioning Engineers.

Austin JB, Russell G (1997). Wheeze, cough, atopy, and indoor environment in the Scottish Highlands. *Archives of Disease in Childhood*, 76:22–26.

Autrup JL et al. (1991). Determination of exposure to aflatoxins among Danish workers in animal-feed production through the analysis of aflatoxin B1 adducts to serum albumin. *Scandinavian Journal of Work, Environment and Health*, 17, 436–440.

Backman E et al. (2000). The effect of air leakage through the moisture damaged structures in a school building having mechanical exhaust ventilation. In: *Proceedings of Healthy Buildings 2000. Vol.3*. Espoo, Sisällmastoseminaarit :141–146.

Baker D, Henderson J (1999). Differences between infants and adults in the social aetiology of wheeze. The ALSPAC Study Team. Avon Longitudinal Study of Pregnancy and Childhood. *Journal of Epidemiology and Community Health* 53:636–642.

Bakke JV et al. (2007). Pet keeping and dampness in the dwelling: associations with airway infections, symptoms, and physiological signs from the ocular and nasal mucosa. *Indoor Air*, 17:60–69.

Bang FB (1956). A bacterial disease of *Limulus polyphemus*. *Bulletin of the John Hopkins Hospital*, 98:325–350.

Barnes C et al. (2006). Comparison of enzyme immunoassay-based assays for environmental *Alternaria alternata*. *Annals of Allergy, Asthma and Immunology*, 97:350–356.

Beijer L, Thorn J, Rylander R (1998). Inhalation of (1→3)-β-D-glucan in humans. In: Wakelyn PJ, Jacobs RR, Rylander R, eds. *Proceedings of the 22nd Cotton and Other Organic Dusts Research Conference*. Memphis, National Research Council:251–253.

Belanger K et al. (2003). Symptoms of wheeze and persistent cough in the first year of life: associations with indoor allergens, air contaminants, and maternal history of asthma. *American Journal of Epidemiology*, 158:195–202.

Belmadani A et al. (1999). Selective toxicity of ochratoxin A in primary cultures from different brain regions. *Archives of Toxicology*, 73:108–114.

Bernstein JA et al. (2006). Health effects of ultraviolet irradiation in asthmatic children's homes. *Journal of Asthma*, 43:255–262.

Biagini JM et al. (2006). Environmental risk factors of rhinitis in early infancy. *Pediatric Allergy and Immunology*, 17:278–284.

Bischof W et al. (2002). Predictors of high endotoxin concentrations in the settled dust of German homes. *Indoor Air*, 12:2–9.

Bloom E et al. (2007). Mass spectrometry-based strategy for direct detection and quantification of some mycotoxins produced by *Stachybotrys* and *Aspergillus* spp. in indoor environments. *Applied and Environmental Microbiology*, 73:4211–4217.

Bolte G et al. (2003). Early endotoxin exposure and atopy development in infants: results of a birth cohort study. *Clinical and Experimental Allergy*, 33:770–776.

Bomberg M, Brown W (1993). Building envelope and environmental control: part 1 — heat, air and moisture interactions. *Construction Canada*, 35:15–18.

Bønløkke JH et al. (2006). Upper-airway inflammation in relation to dust spiked with aldehydes or glucan. *Scandinavian Journal of Work, Environment and Health*, 32:374–382.

Bonner S et al. (2006). Self-reported moisture or mildew in the homes of Head Start children with asthma is associated with greater asthma morbidity. *Journal of Urban Health*, 83:129–137.

Bornehag CG et al. (2001). Dampness in buildings and health: Nordic interdisciplinary review of the scientific evidence on associations between exposure to 'dampness' in buildings and health effects (NORDDAMP). *Indoor Air*, 11:72–86.

Bornehag CG et al. (2004). Dampness in buildings as a risk factor for health effects, EUROEXPO: a multidisciplinary review of the literature (1998–2000) on dampness and mite exposure in buildings and health effects. *Indoor Air*, 14:243–257.

Bornehag CG et al. (2005). 'Dampness' at home and its association with airway, nose, and skin symptoms among 10,851 preschool children in Sweden: a cross-sectional study. *Indoor Air*, 15(Suppl. 10):48–55.

Bottcher MF et al. (2003). Endotoxin levels in Estonian and Swedish house dust and atopy in infancy. *Clinical and Experimental Allergy*, 33:295–300.

Bouillard LA, Devleeschouwer MJ, Michel O (2006). Characteristics of the home bacterial contamination and endotoxin related release. *Journal de Pharmacie de Belgique*, 61:63–66.

Brasel TL et al. (2005a). Detection of airborne *Stachybotrys chartarum* macrocyclic trichothecene mycotoxins in the indoor environment. *Applied and Environmental Microbiology*, 71:7376–7388.

Brasel TL et al. (2005b). Detection of airborne *Stachybotrys chartarum* macrocyclic trichothecene mycotoxins on particulates smaller than conidia. *Applied and Environmental Microbiology*, 71:114–122.

Braun-Fahrländer C (2003). Environmental exposure to endotoxin and other microbial products and the decreased risk of childhood atopy: evaluating developments since April 2002. *Current Opinion in Allergy and Clinical Immunology*, 3:325–329.

Braun-Fahrländer C et al. (2002). Environmental exposure to endotoxin and its relation to asthma in school-age children. *New England Journal of Medicine*, 347:869–877.

Brunekreef B (1992). Damp housing and adult respiratory symptoms. *Allergy*, 47:498–502.

Brunekreef B et al. (1989). Home dampness and respiratory morbidity in children. *American Review of Respiratory Diseases*, 140:1363–1367.

Bryant DH, Rogers P (1991). Allergic alveolitis due to wood-rot fungi. *Allergy Proceedings*, 12:89–94.

Burch DM, Saunders CA (1995). *A computer analysis of wall constructions in the moisture control handbook*. Gaithersburg, Building and Fire Research Laboratory, National Institute of Standards and Technology.

Burke S, Yverås V (2004). A Swedish perspective on the prevention of moisture problems during the building's design phase. *Nordic Journal of Surveying and Real Estate Research*, 1:102–113.

Bush RK, Prochnau JJ (2004). Alternaria-induced asthma. *Journal of Allergy and Clinical Immunology*, 113:227–234.

Bush RK et al. (2006). The medical effects of mold exposure. *Journal of Allergy and Clinical Immunology*, 117:326–333.

CEN (2007a). *European Standard EN 13779. Ventilation for non-residential buildings - performance requirements for ventilation and room-conditioning systems*. Brussels, European Committee for Standardization.

CEN (2007b). *European Standard EN15251. Indoor environmental input parameters for design and assessment of energy performance of buildings addressing indoor air quality, thermal environment, lighting and acoustics*. Brussels, European Committee for Standardization.

Centers for Disease Control and Prevention (1994). Acute pulmonary hemorrhage/hemosiderosis among infants — Cleveland, January 1993–November 1994. *Morbidity and Mortality Weekly Report*, 43:881–883.

Centers for Disease Control and Prevention (1997). Update: pulmonary hemor-rhage/hemosiderosis among infants — Cleveland, Ohio, 1993–1996. *Morbidity and Mortality Weekly Report*, 46:33–35.

Centers for Disease Control and Prevention (2000). Update: pulmonary hemor-rhage/hemosiderosis among infants — Cleveland, Ohio, 1993–1996. *Morbidity and Mortality Weekly Report*, 49:180–184.

Cerny R, Madera J, Grunewald J (2001). Numerical simulation of heat and mois-ture transport in building envelopes with inside thermal insulation systems on the mineral wool basic. In: *Proceedings of the International Conference on Building Envelope Systems and Technologies, Ottawa, 26–29 June 2001*. Ottawa, National Research Council, Institute for Research in Construction:251–255.

Charpin-Kadouch C et al. (2006). Mycotoxin identification in moldy dwellings. *Journal of Applied Toxicology*, 26:475–479.

Chen CM et al. (2007). Social factors, allergen, endotoxin, and dust mass in mat-tress. *Indoor Air*, 17:384–393.

Chew GL et al. (2001). Fungal extracellular polysaccharides, beta (1→3)-glucans and culturable fungi in repeated sampling of house dust. *Indoor Air*, 11:171–178.

Cho S et al. (2005). Aerodynamic characteristics and respiratory deposition of fungal fragments. *Atmospheric Environment*, 39:5454–5465.

Cho SH et al. (2006). Mold damage in homes and wheezing in infants. *Annals of Allergy, Asthma and Immunology*, 97:539–545.

Chun DT et al. (2000). Preliminary report on the results of the second phase of a round-robin endotoxin assay study using cotton dust. *Applied Occupational and Environmental Hygiene*, 15:152–157.

Chung YJ et al. (2005). Dose-dependent allergic responses to an extract of *Penicillium chrysogenum* in BALB/c mice. *Toxicology*, 209:77–89.

Claeson AS, Sandstrom M, Sunesson AL (2007). Volatile organic compounds (VOCs) emitted from materials collected from buildings affected by microor-ganisms. *Journal of Environmental Monitoring*, 9:240–245.

Cochran WG (1968). Errors of measurement in statistics. *Technometrics*, 10:637–666.

Cormier Y, Belanger J (1989). The fluctuant nature of precipitating antibodies in dairy farmers. *Thorax*, 44:469–473.

Cuijpers CE et al. (1995). Adverse effects of the indoor environment on respira-tory health in primary school children. *Environmental Research*, 68:11–23.

Dales RE, Miller D (1999). Residential fungal contamination and health: micro-bial cohabitants as covariates. *Environmental Health Perspectives*, 107(Suppl. 3):481–483.

Dales RE, Burnett R, Zwanenburg H (1991). Adverse health effects among adults exposed to home dampness and molds. *American Review of Respiratory Dis-eases*, 143:505–509.

Dales RE, Miller D, McMullen E (1997). Indoor air quality and health: validity and determinants of reported home dampness and moulds. *International Journal of Epidemiology*, 26:120–125.

Dales RE, Miller D, White J (1999). Testing the association between residential fungus and health using ergosterol measures and cough recordings. *Mycopathologia*, 147:21–27.

Dales R et al. (2006). Airborne endotoxin is associated with respiratory illness in the first 2 years of life. *Environmental Health Perspectives*, 114:610–614.

de Andrade AD et al. (1995). House dust mite allergen content in two areas with large differences in relative humidity. *Annals of Allergy, Asthma and Immunology*, 74:314–316.

Dekker C et al. (1991). Childhood asthma and the indoor environment. *Chest*, 100:922–926.

DeKoster JA, Thorne PS (1995). Bioaerosol concentrations in noncomplaint, complaint and intervention homes in the Midwest. *American Industrial Hygiene Association Journal*, 56:573–580.

Dharmage S et al. (2001). Current indoor allergen levels of fungi and cats, but not house dust mites, influence allergy and asthma in adults with high dust mite exposure. *American Journal of Respiratory and Critical Care Medicine*, 164:65–71.

Dharmage S et al. (2002). Mouldy houses influence symptoms of asthma among atopic individuals. *Clinical and Experimental Allergy*, 32:714–720.

Dijkstra L et al. (1990). Respiratory health effects of the indoor environment in a population of Dutch children. *American Review of Respiratory Diseases*, 142:1172–1178.

Dillon HK, Heinsohn PA, Miller JD, eds (1996). *Field guide for the determination of biological contaminants in environmental samples*. Fairfax, VA, American Industrial Hygiene Association.

Donohue M et al. (2006). Characterization of nigerlysin, hemolysin produced by *Aspergillus niger*, and effect on mouse neuronal cells in vitro. *Toxicology*, 219:150–155.

Dotterud LK, Falk ES (1999). Atopic disease among adults in Northern Russia, an area with heavy air pollution. *Acta Dermato-Venereologica*, 79:448–450.

Douwes J (2005). (1→3)-beta-D-glucans and respiratory health: a review of the scientific evidence. *Indoor Air*, 15:160–169.

Douwes J, Pearce N, Heederik D (2002). Does environmental endotoxin exposure prevent asthma? *Thorax*, 57:86–90.

Douwes J et al. (1995). Influence of various dust sampling and extraction methods on the measurement of airborne endotoxin. *Applied and Environmental Microbiology*, 61:1763–1769.

Douwes J et al. (1996). Measurement of β(1→3)-glucans in the occupational and home environment with an inhibition enzyme immunoassay. *Applied and Environmental Microbiology*, 62:3176–3182.

Douwes J et al. (1998). Endotoxin and β(1→3)-glucan in house dust and the relation with home characteristics: a pilot study in 25 German houses. *Indoor Air*, 8:255–263.

Douwes J et al. (1999). Fungal extracellular polysaccharides in house dust as a marker for exposure to fungi: relations with culturable fungi, reported home dampness, and respiratory symptoms. *Journal of Allergy and Clinical Immunology*, 103:494–500.

Douwes J et al. (2000). (1→3)-β-D-glucan and endotoxin in house dust and peak flow variability in children. *American Journal of Respiratory and Critical Care Medicine*, 162:1348–1354.

Douwes J et al. (2004). Can bacterial endotoxin exposure reverse atopy and atopic disease? *Journal of Allergy and Clinical Immunology*, 114:1051–1054.

Douwes J et al. (2006). Does early indoor microbial exposure reduce the risk of asthma? The Prevention and Incidence of Asthma and Mite Allergy birth cohort study. *Journal of Allergy and Clinical Immunology*, 117:1067–1073.

Duchaine C et al. (2001). Comparison of endotoxin exposure assessment by bioaerosol impinger and filter sampling methods. *Applied and Environmental Microbiology*, 67:2775–2780.

Dufour X et al. (2006). Paranasal sinus fungus ball: epidemiology, clinical features and diagnosis. A retrospective analysis of 173 cases from a single medical center in France, 1989–2002. *Medical Mycology*, 44:61–67.

du Prel X, Kramer U, Ranft U (2005). Changes in social inequality with respect to health-related living conditions of 6-year-old children in East Germany after re-unification. *BMC Public Health*, 5:64.

du Prel X et al. (2006). Preschool children's health and its association with parental education and individual living conditions in East and West Germany. *BMC Public Health*, 6:312.

Ebbehoj NE et al. (2005). Molds in floor dust, building-related symptoms, and lung function among male and female schoolteachers. *Indoor Air*, 15(Suppl. 10):7–16.

Eduard W (2006). Fungal spores. The Nordic Expert Group for Criteria Documentation of Health Risk from Chemicals. *Arbete och Hälsa*, 21:1–145.

Eduard W, Heederik D (1998). Methods for quantitative assessment of airborne levels of non-infectious microorganisms in highly contaminated work environments. *American Industrial Hygiene Association Journal*, 59:113–127.

Eduard W et al. (1988). Identification and quantification of mould spores by scanning electron microscopy (SEM): analysis of filter samples collected in Norwegian saw mills. *Annals of Occupational Hygiene*, 31(Suppl. 1):447–455.

Eduard W et al. (2001). Short term exposure to airborne microbial agents during farm work: exposure–response relations with eye and respiratory symptoms. *Occupational and Environmental Medicine*, 58:113–118.

Ehrlich K (1987). Effect on aflatoxin production of competition between wild-type and mutant strains of *Aspergillus parasiticus. Mycopathologia*, 97:93–96.

El Sharif N et al. (2004). Concentrations of domestic mite and pet allergens and endotoxin in Palestine. *Allergy*, 59:623–631.

Emenius G et al. (2004a). Building characteristics, indoor air quality and recurrent wheezing in very young children (BAMSE). *Indoor Air*, 14:34–42.

Emenius G et al. (2004b). Indoor exposures and recurrent wheezing in infants: a study in the BAMSE cohort. *Acta Paediatrica*, 93:899–905.

Engman LH, Bornehag CG, Sundell J (2007). How valid are parents' questionnaire responses regarding building characteristics, mouldy odour, and signs of moisture problems in Swedish homes? *Scandinavian Journal of Public Health*, 35:125–132.

Engvall K, Norrby C, Norbäck D (2001). Asthma symptoms in relation to building dampness and odour in older multifamily houses in Stockholm. *International Journal of Tuberculosis and Lung Disease*, 5:468–477.

Engvall K, Norrby C, Norbäck D (2002). Ocular, airway, and dermal symptoms related to building dampness and odors in dwellings. *Archives of Environmental Health*, 57:304–310.

Etzel RA et al. (1998). Acute pulmonary hemorrhage in infants associated with exposure to *Stachybotrys atra* and other fungi. *Archives of Pediatric and Adolescent Medicine*, 152:757–762.

European Collaborative Action on Urban Air, Indoor Environment and Human Health (2003). *Ventilation, good indoor air quality and rational use of energy.* Ispra, European Commission, Joint Research Centre, Institute for Health and Human Protection, Physical and Chemical Exposure Unit (Report No. 23).

Fanger PO (1988). Introduction of the olf and the decipol units to quantify air pollution perceived by humans indoors and outdoors. *Energy and Buildings*, 12:1–6.

Fergusson RJ, Milne LJ, Crompton GK (1984). Penicillium allergic alveolitis: faulty installation of central heating. *Thorax*, 39:294–298.

Finnish Society of Indoor Air Quality and Climate (2001). *Classification of indoor climate 2000.* Espoo, Finnish Society of Indoor Air Quality and Climate (Publication 5 E).

Fisk WJ, Lei-Gomez Q, Mendell MJ (2007). Meta-analyses of the associations of respiratory health effects with dampness and mold in homes. *Indoor Air*, 17:284–296Fisk WJ et al. (2002). Performance and costs of particle air filtration technologies. *Indoor Air*, 12:223–234.

Fitzpatrick FA (2001). Inflammation, carcinogenesis and cancer. *International Immunopharmacology*, 1:1651–1667.

Flannigan B, Morey P (1996). *Control of moisture problems affecting biological indoor air quality. ISIAQ guideline*. Ottawa, International Society of Indoor Air and Climate.

Flannigan B, Samson RA, Miller JD, eds (2001). *Microorganisms in home and indoor work environments*. New York, Taylor & Francis.

Flemming J, Hudson B, Rand TG (2004). Comparison of inflammatory and cytotoxic lung responses in mice after intratracheal exposure to spores of two different *Stachybotrys chartarum* strains. *Toxicological Sciences*, 78:267–275.

Fogelmark B, Sjöstrand M, Rylander R (1994). Pulmonary inflammation induced by repeated inhalations of β(1,3)-D-glucan and endotoxin. *International Journal of Experimental Pathology*, 75:85–90.

Fogelmark B, Thorn J, Rylander R (2001). Inhalation of (1→3)-β-D-glucan causes airway eosinophilia. *Mediators of Inflammation*, 10:13–19.

Fogelmark B et al. (1992). Acute pulmonary toxicity of inhaled β-1,3-glucan and endotoxin. *Agents and Actions*, 35:50–56.

Forsberg B et al. (1997). Childhood asthma in four regions in Scandinavia: risk factors and avoidance effects. *International Journal of Epidemiology*, 26:610–619.

Foto M (2004). Modification of the *Limulus* amebocyte lysate assay for the analysis of glucan in indoor environments. *Analytical and Bioanalytical Chemistry*, 379:156–162.

Gallup J et al. (1987). Indoor mold spore exposure: characteristics of 127 homes in southern California with endogenous mold problems. *Experientia*, 51(Suppl.):139–142.

Garrett MH, Rayment PR, Hooper MJ (1998). Indoor fungal spores, house dampness and associations with environmental factors and respiratory health in children. *Clinical and Experimental Allergy*, 28:459–467.

Gehring U et al. (2001). β(1→3)-glucan in house dust of German homes related to culturable mold spore counts, housing and occupant characteristics. *Environmental Health Perspectives*, 109:139–144.

Gehring U et al. (2002). House dust endotoxin and allergic sensitization in children. *American Journal of Respiratory and Critical Care Medicine*, 166:939–944.

Geisler WM, Corey L (2002). *Chlamydia pneumoniae* respiratory infection after allogeneic stem cell transplantation. *Transplantation*, 73:1002–1005.

Gent JF et al. (2002). Levels of household mold associated with respiratory symptoms in the first year of life in a cohort at risk for asthma. *Environmental Health Perspectives*, 110:A781–A786.

Gereda JE et al. (2000). Relation between house-dust endotoxin exposure, type 1 T-cell development, and allergen sensitisation in infants at high risk of asthma. *Lancet*, 355:1680–1683.

Giovannangelo M et al. (2007). Determinants of house dust endotoxin in three European countries – the AIRALLERG study. *Indoor Air*, 17:70–79.

Godish T, Rouch J (1986). Mitigation of residential formaldehyde contamination by indoor climate control. *American Industrial Hygiene Association Journal*, 47:792–797.

Goebes MD et al. (2007). Real-time PCR for detection of the *Aspergillus* genus. *Journal of Environmental Monitoring*, 9:599–609.

Gorny RL (2004). Filamentous microorganisms and their fragments in indoor air – a review. *Annals of Agricultural and Environmental Medicine*, 11:185–197.

Gorny RL, Dutkiewicz J, Krysinska-Traczyk E (1999). Size distribution of bacterial and fungal bioaerosols in indoor air. *Annals of Agricultural and Environmental Medicine*, 6:105–113.

Gorny RL et al. (2002). Fungal fragments as indoor air biocontaminants. *Applied and Environmental Microbiology*, 68:3522–3531.

Grant C et al. (1989). The moisture requirements of moulds isolated from domestic dwellings. *International Biodeterioration and Biodegradation*, 25:259–284.

Gravesen S, Frisvad JC, Samson RA (1994). *Microfungi*. Copenhagen, Munksgaard.

Green BJ et al. (2006). Airborne fungal fragments and allergenicity. *Medical Mycology*, 44(Suppl. 1):S245–S255.

Gregory L et al. (2003). Immunocytochemical localization of stachylysin in *Stachybotrys chartarum* spores and spore-impacted mouse and rat lung tissue. *Mycopathologia*, 156:109–117.

Gunnbjörnsdóttir MI et al. (2003). The relationship between indicators of building dampness and respiratory health in young Swedish adults. *Respiratory Medicine*, 97:302–307.

Gunnbjörnsdóttir MI et al. (2006). Prevalence and incidence of respiratory symptoms in relation to indoor dampness: the RHINE study. *Thorax*, 61:221–225.

Hänninen OO et al. (2004). Infiltration of ambient PM2.5 and levels of indoor generated non-ETS PM2.5 in residences of four European cities. *Atmospheric Environment*, 38: 6411–6423.

Hänninen O et al. (2005). Reduction potential of urban $PM_{2.5}$ mortality risk using modern ventilation systems in buildings. *Indoor Air*, 15:246–256.

Hansen JS et al. (2007). Adjuvant effects of inhaled mono-2-ethylhexyl phthalate in BALB/cJ mice. *Toxicology*, 232:79–88.

Hardin BD, Kelman BJ, Saxon A (2003). Adverse human health effects associated with molds in the indoor environment. *Journal of Occupational and Environmental Medicine*, 45:470–478.

Häupl P, Fechnerm H (2003). Moisture behaviour within the 'Church of Our Lady' in Dresden, Germany. In: Hens H, Vermeir G, Carmeliet J, eds. *Research in building physics*. Lisse, Balkema:785–792.

Häupl P, Jurk K, Petzold H (2003). Inside thermal insulation for historical facades. In: Hens H, Vermeir G, Carmeliet J, eds. *Research in building physics.*
Lisse, Balkema:463–470.

Haverinen U (2002). *Modeling moisture damage observations and their association with health symptoms* [thesis]. Kuopio, National Public Health Institute, Department of Environmental Health, University of Kuopio (Report
A10/2002).

Haverinen U et al. (2001). Comparison of two-level and three-level classifica-
tions of moisture-damaged dwellings in relation to health effects. *Indoor Air,*
11:192–199.

Haverinen-Shaughnessy U et al.(2007). Personal and microenvironmental concentrations of particles and microbial aerosol in relation to health symptoms
among teachers. *Journal of Exposure Science and Environmental Epidemiology,*
17:182–190.

Heederik D, Attfield M (2000). Characterization of dust exposure for the study of
chronic occupational lung disease: a comparison of different exposure assessment strategies. *American Journal of Epidemiology,* 151:982–990.

Heederik D, Douwes J, Thorne PS (2003). Biological agents — evaluation. In:
Perkins J, ed. *Modern industrial hygiene,* Vol. 2. Cincinnati, American Conference of Governmental Industrial Hygienists.

Heldal KK et al. (2003). Upper airway inflammation in waste handlers exposed
to bioaerosols. *Occupational and Environmental Medicine,* 60:444–450.

Hersoug LG (2005). Viruses as the causative agent related to 'dampness' and the
missing link between allergen exposure and onset of allergic disease. *Indoor
Air,* 15:363–366.

Hirvonen MR et al. (1999). Nitric oxide and proinflammatory cytokines in nasal
lavage fluid associated with symptoms and exposure to moldy building microbes. *American Journal of Respiratory and Critical Care Medicine,* 160:1943–
1946.

Hirvonen MR et al. (2001). *Streptomyces anulatus* induced inflammatory responses and cytotoxicity in macrophages are regulated by growth conditions
of the microbe. *Inhalation Toxicology,* 13:55–68.

Hollander A, Heederik D, Doekes G (1997). Respiratory allergy to rats: exposure–response relationships in laboratory animal workers. *American Journal
of Critical Care Medicine,* 155:562–567.

Hope AP, Simon RA (2007). Excess dampness and mold growth in homes: an
evidence-based review of the aeroirritant effect and its potential causes. *Allergy and Asthma Proceedings,* 28:262–270.

Hu FB et al. (1997). An epidemiological study of asthma prevalence and related
factors among young adults. *Journal of Asthma,* 34:67–76.

Hunter CA et al. (1988). Mould in buildings: the air spora of domestic dwellings.
International Biodeterioration and Biodegradation, 24:81–101.

Huttunen K et al. (2000). Inflammatory responses in RAW264.7 macrophages caused by mycobacteria isolated from moldy houses. *Environmental Toxicology and Pharmacology*, 8:237–244.

Huttunen K et al. (2001). Comparison of mycobacteria-induced cytotoxicity and inflammatory responses in human and mouse cell lines. *Inhalation Toxicology*, 13:977–991.

Huttunen K et al. (2003). Production of proinflammatory mediators by indoor air bacteria and fungal spores in mouse and human cell lines. *Environmental Health Perspectives*, 111:85–92.

Huttunen K et al. (2004). Synergistic interaction in simultaneous exposure to *Streptomyces californicus* and *Stachybotrys chartarum*. *Environmental Health Perspectives*, 112:659–665.

Hyvärinen A et al. (2002). Fungi and actinobacteria in moisture-damaged building materials – concentrations and diversity. *International Biodeterioration and Biodegradation*, 49:27–37.

IARC (1993). *IARC monographs on the evaluation of carcinogenic risks to humans. Vol. 56: Some naturally occurring substances: food items and constituents, heterocyclic aromatic amines and mycotoxins – summary of data reported and evaluation.* Lyon, International Agency for Research on Cancer:245–489.

Immonen J et al. (2001). Skin-prick test findings in students from moisture- and mold-damaged schools: a 3-year follow-up study. *Pediatric Allergy and Immunology*, 12:87–94.

Infante-Rivard C (1993). Childhood asthma and indoor environmental risk factors. *American Journal of Epidemiology*, 137:834–844.

Institute of Medicine (2000). *Clearing the air: asthma and indoor air exposures.* Washington, DC, National Academies Press.

Institute of Medicine (2004) *Damp indoor spaces and health.* Washington, DC, National Academies Press.

ISIAQ (1996). *TFI-1119, Control of moisture problems affecting biological indoor air quality.* Espoo, International Society of Indoor Air Quality and Climate (ISIAQ guideline, task force 1-1996; http://www.isiaq.org/publication.asp, accessed 12 May 2009).

Iossifova YY et al. (2007). House dust (1→3)- β-D-glucan and wheezing in infants. *Allergy*, 62:504–513.

Islam Z, Harkema JR, Pestka JJ (2006). Satratoxin G from the black mold *Stachybotrys chartarum* evokes olfactory sensory neuron loss and inflammation in the murine nose and brain. *Environmental Health Perspectives*, 114:1099–1107.

Islam Z et al. (2007). Neurotoxicity and inflammation in the nasal airways of mice exposed to the macrocyclic trichothecene mycotoxin roridin A: kinetics and potentiation by bacterial lipopolysaccharide coexposure. *Toxicological Sciences*, 98:526–541.

Iversen M et al. (1990). Mite allergy and exposure to storage mites and house dust mites in farmers. *Clinical and Experimental Allergy*, 20:211–219.

Iwen PC et al. (1994). Airborne fungal spore monitoring in a protective environment during hospital construction, and correlation with an outbreak of invasive aspergillosis. *Infection Control and Hospital Epidemiology*, 15:303–306.

Iwen PC et al. (1998) Invasive pulmonary aspergillosis due to *Aspergillus terreus*: 12-year experience and review of the literature. *Clinical Infectious Diseases*, 26:1092–1097.

Jaakkola JJ, Jaakkola N, Ruotsalainen R (1993). Home dampness and molds as determinants of respiratory symptoms and asthma in pre-school children. *Journal of Exposure Analysis and Environmental Epidemiology*, 3(Suppl.1):129–142.

Jaakkola JJ, Hwang BF, Jaakkola N (2005). Home dampness and molds, parental atopy, and asthma in childhood: a six-year population-based cohort study. *Environmental Health Perspectives*, 113:357–361.

Jaakkola MS et al. (2002). Indoor dampness and molds and development of adult-onset asthma: a population-based incident case-control study. *Environmental Health Perspectives*, 110:543–547.

Jacob B et al. (2002). Indoor exposure to molds and allergic sensitisation. *Environmental Health Perspectives*, 110:647–653.

Janssen NAH et al. (1999). Personal exposure to fine particles in children correlates closely with ambient fine particles. *Archives of Environmental Health*, 54:95–101.

Janssen NAH et al. (2000). Personal exposure to fine particulate matter in elderly subjects: relation between personal, indoor, and outdoor concentrations. *Journal of the Air and Waste Management Association*, 50:1133–1143.

Janssen NAH et al. (2002). Air conditioning and source-specific particles as modifiers of the effect of PM10 on hospital admissions for heart and lung disease. *Environmental Health Perspectives*, 110:43–49.

Janssens A, Hens H (2003). Interstitial condensation due to air leakage: a sensitivity analysis. *Journal of Thermal Envelope and Building Science*, 27:15–29.

Jędrychowski W, Flak E (1998). Separate and combined effects of the outdoor and indoor air quality on chronic respiratory symptoms adjusted for allergy among preadolescent children. *International Journal of Occupational Medicine and Environmental Health*, 11:19–35.

Johannessen LN, Nilsen AM, Lovik M (2005). The mycotoxins citrinin and gliotoxin differentially affect production of the pro-inflammatory cytokines tumour necrosis factor-α and interleukin-6, and the anti-inflammatory cytokine interleukin-10. *Clinical and Experimental Allergy*, 35:782–789.

Johannessen LN, Nilsen AM, Lovik M (2007). Mycotoxin-induced depletion of intracellular glutathione and altered cytokine production in the human alveolar epithelial cell line A549. *Toxicological Letters*, 168:103–112.

Johanning E et al. (1996). Health and immunology study following exposure to toxigenic fungi (*Stachybotrys chartarum*) in a water-damaged office environment. *International Archives of Occupational and Environmental Health*, 68:207–218.

Johansson P et al. (2005). *Microbiological growth on building materials – critical moisture levels. State of the art.* Borås, SP Swedish National Testing and Research Institute (Report 2005:11; http://www.kuleuven.ac.be/bwf/projects/annex41/protected/data/SP%20Oct%202005%20Prese%20A41-T4-S-05-7.pdf, accessed 16 March 2009).

Jovanovic S et al. (2004). Indoor fungi levels in homes of children with and without allergy history. *International Journal of Hygiene and Environmental Health*, 207:369–378.

Jussila J et al. (1999). *Streptomyces anulatus* from indoor air of moldy houses induce NO and IL-6 production in a human alveolar epithelial cell-line. *Environmental Toxicology and Pharmacology*, 7:261–266.

Jussila J et al. (2001). Inflammatory responses in mice after intratracheal instillation of spores of *Streptomyces californicus* isolated from indoor air of a moldy building. *Toxicology and Applied Pharmacology*, 171:61–69.

Jussila J et al. (2002a). *Mycobacterium terrae* isolated from indoor air of a moisture-damaged building induces sustained biphasic inflammatory response in mouse lungs. *Environmental Health Perspectives*, 110:1119–1125.

Jussila J et al. (2002b). Inflammatory potential of the spores of *Penicillium spinulosum* isolated from indoor air of a moisture-damaged building in mouse lungs. *Environmental Toxicology and Pharmacology*, 12:137–145.

Jussila J et al. (2002c). Spores of *Aspergillus versicolor* isolated from indoor air of a moisture-damaged building provoke acute inflammation in mouse lungs. *Inhalation Toxicology*, 14:1261–1277.

Jussila J et al. (2003). Systemic immunoresponses in mice after repeated exposure of lungs to spores of *Streptomyces californicus*. *Clinical and Diagnostic Laboratory Immunology*, 10:30–37.

Kalagasidis AS, Mattsson B (2005). Modelling of moisture conditions in a cold attic space. In: *Ventilation in relation to the energy performance of buidlings. Conference report.* Brussels, Air Infiltration and Ventilation Centre:53–58.

Kalamees T (2006). *Hygrothermal criteria for design and simulation of buildings* [thesis]. Tallinn, Tallinn University of Technology.

Kalamees T et al. (2007). Air pressure conditions in Finnish residences. In: Seppänen O, Säteri J, eds. *Clima 2007: WellBeing Indoors* [CD-ROM]. Helsinki, Finnish Association of HVAC Societies.

Kamp HG et al. (2005). Ochratoxin A: induction of (oxidative) DNA damage, cytotoxicity and apoptosis in mammalian cell lines and primary cells. *Toxicology*, 206:413–425.

Karagiozis A (2002). *Building enclosure hygrothermal performance study phase I.* Oak Ridge, Oak Ridge National Laboratory (Report No. ORNL/TM-2002/89).

Karevold G et al. (2006). Respiratory infections in schoolchildren: co-morbidity and risk factors. *Archives of Disease in Childhood*, 91:391–395.

Karlsson K, Malmberg P (1989). Characterization of exposure to molds and actinomycetes in agricultural dusts by scanning electron microscopy, fluorescence microscopy and the culture method. *Scandinavian Journal of Work, Environment and Health*, 15:353–359.

Kauffman HF (2003). Immunopathogenesis of allergic bronchopulmonary aspergillosis and airway remodeling. *Frontiers in Bioscience*, 8:e190–e196.

Kercsmar CM et al. (2006). Reduction in asthma morbidity in children as a result of home remediation aimed at moisture sources. *Environmental Health Perspectives*, 114:1574–1580.

Khan AA, Cerniglia CE (1994). Detection of *Pseudomonas aeruginosa* from clinical and environmental samples by amplification of the exotoxin A gene using PCR. *Applied and Environmental Microbiology*, 60: 3739–3745.

Kilpeläinen M et al. (2000). Heat and moisture distribution at the connection of floor and external wall in multi-storey timber frame houses. In: *Proceedings of the 6th World Conference on Timber Engineering, Whistler Resort, British Columbia* [CD-ROM]. Vancouver, Canadian Pension and Benefits Institute.

Kilpeläinen M et al. (2001). Home dampness, current allergic diseases, and respiratory infections among young adults. *Thorax*, 56:462–467.

Klis FM (1994). Review: cell wall assembly in yeast. *Yeast*, 10:851–869.

Kolstad HA et al. (2002). Do indoor molds in nonindustrial environments threaten workers' health? A review of the epidemiologic evidence. *Epidemiologic Reviews*, 24:203–217.

Koskinen OM et al. (1999a). Adverse health effects in children associated with moisture and mold observations in houses. *International Journal of Environmental Health Research*, 9:143–156.

Koskinen OM et al. (1999b). The relationship between moisture or mould observations in houses and the state of health of their occupants. *European Respiratory Journal*, 14:1363–1367.

Kreiss K (1989). The epidemiology of building-related complaints and illness. *Occupational Medicine*, 4:575–592.

Kristensen P, Andersen A, Irgens LM (2000). Hormone-dependent cancer and adverse reproductive outcomes in farmers' families – effects of climatic conditions favoring fungal growth in grain. *Scandinavian Journal of Work, Environment and Health*, 26:331–337.

Krus M, Sedlbauer K (2002). Brauchen wir Gefährdungsklassen für Schimmelpilze zur Beurteilung von Baukonstruktionen? In: *11. Bauklimatisches Symposium 2002. Tagungsbeiträge, Dresden, 26–30 September 2002*. Vol. 2. Dresden, Institut für Bauklimatik, Technische Universität:790–802.

Krus M, Sedlbauer K. (2007). A new model for prediction and its application in practice. In: *Proceedings of the 6th International Conference on Indoor Air Quality, Ventilation and Energy Conservation in Buildings, Sendai, Japan, 28–31 October 2007* [CD-ROM]. Brussels, Air Infilitration and Ventilation Centre.

Kurnitski J (2000a). Crawl space air change, heat and moisture behaviour. *Energy and Buildings*, 32:19–39.

Kurnitski J (2000b). *Humidity control in outdoor-air-ventilated crawl spaces in cold climate by means of ventilation, ground covers and dehumidification* [thesis]. Espoo, Helsinki University of Technology, Department of Mechanical Engineering, Laboratory of Heating, Ventilating and Air Conditioning (Report A3).

Kurnitski J (2006). Pientalojen ilmanvaihto ja ilmanpitävyys [Ventilation and air tightness in houses]. In: Koskenvesa A et al., eds. *Rakentajain kalenteri [Builders' Yearbook]*, Helsinki, Rakennustieto Oy: 415–424

Kurnitski J, Pasanen P (2000). Crawl space moisture and microbes. In: *Proceedings of Healthy Buildings 2000*. Vol.3. Espoo, Sisällmastoseminaarit:205–210.

Kurnitski J et al. (2007). Potential effects of permeable and hygroscopic lightweight structures on thermal comfort and perceived IAQ in a cold climate. *Indoor Air*, 17:37–49.

Kuyucu S et al. (2006). Epidemiologic characteristics of rhinitis in Turkish children: the International Study of Asthma and Allergies in Childhood (ISAAC) phase 2. *Pediatric Allergy and Immunology*, 17:269–277.

Kwon OS, Slikker W Jr, Davies DL (2000). Biochemical and morphological effects of fumonisin B(1) on primary cultures of rat cerebrum. *Neurotoxicology and Teratology*, 22:565–572.

Lange JH (2004). Endotoxin as a factor for joint pain and rheumatoid arthritis. *Clinical Rheumatology*, 23:566.

Lange JL, Thorne PS, Lynch NL (1997). Application of flow cytometry and fluorescent in situ hybridization for assessment of exposures to airborne bacteria. *Applied and Environmental Microbiology*, 63:1557–1563.

Larsen FO et al. (1996). Microfungi in indoor air are able to trigger histamine release by non-IgE-mediated mechanisms. *Inflammation Research*, 45:S23–S24.

Lawson JA et al. (2005). Regional variations in risk factors for asthma in school children. *Canadian Respiratory Journal*, 12:321–326.

Leaderer BP et al. (2002). Dust mite, cockroach, cat, and dog allergen concentrations in homes of asthmatic children in the northeastern United States: impact of socioeconomic factors and population density. *Environmental Health Perspectives*, 110:419–425.

Ledford DK (1994). Indoor allergens. *Journal of Allergy and Clinical Immunology*, 94:327–334.

Lednicky JA, Rayner JO (2006). Uncommon respiratory pathogens. *Current Opinion in Pulmonary Medicine*, 12:235–239.

Lee YL et al. (2006). Home exposures, parental atopy, and occurrence of asthma symptoms in adulthood in southern Taiwan. *Chest*, 129:300–308.

Leech JA, Raizenne M, Gusdorf J. (2004). Health in occupants of energy efficient new homes. *Indoor Air*, 14:169–173.

Lehtinen T (2000). Thermal and moisture physical design and dimensioning methods of structures. In: *Proceedings of Healthy Buildings 2000*. Vol.3. Espoo, Sisällmastoseminaarit:507–512.

Leino M et al. (2003). Intranasal exposure to a damp building mould, *Stachybotrys chartarum*, induces lung inflammation in mice by satratoxin-independent mechanisms. *Clinical and Experimental Allergy*, 33:1603–1610.

Leino MS et al. (2006). Intranasal exposure to *Stachybotrys chartarum* enhances airway inflammation in allergic mice. *American Journal of Respiratory and Critical Care Medicine*, 173:512–518.

Li CS, Hsu LY (1996). Home dampness and childhood respiratory symptoms in a subtropical climate. *Archives of Environmental Health*, 51:42–46.

Li CS, Hsu LY (1997). Airborne fungus allergen in association with residential characteristics in atopic and control children in a subtropical region. *Archives of Environmental Health*, 52:72–79.

Li CS, Kuo YM (1994). Characteristics of airborne microfungi in subtropical homes. *Science of the Total Environment*, 155:267–271.

Li M et al. (2006). T-2 toxin impairs murine immune response to respiratory reovirus and exacerbates viral bronchiolitis. *Toxicology and Applied Pharmacology*, 217:76–85.

Li M et al. (2007). Deoxynivalenol exacerbates viral bronchopneumonia induced by respiratory reovirus infection. *Toxicological Sciences*, 95:412–426.

Li Y et al. (2007). Role of ventilation in airborne transmission of infectious agents in the built environment — a multidisciplinary systematic review. *Indoor Air*, 17:2–18.

Liu AH (2007). Hygiene theory and allergy and asthma prevention. *Paediatric and Perinatal Epidemiology*, 21(Suppl. 3):2–7.

Liu AH, Leung DY (2006). Renaissance of the hygiene hypothesis. *Journal of Allergy and Clinical Immunology*, 117:1063–1066.

Liu DL, Nazaroff WW (2001). Modeling pollutant penetration across building envelopes. *Atmospheric Environment*, 35:4451–4462.

Liu DL, Nazaroff WW (2003). Particle penetration through building cracks. *Aerosol Science and Technology*, 37:565–573.

Lorenz W et al. (2006). A hypothesis for the origin and pathogenesis of rheumatoid diseases. *Rheumatology International*, 26:641–654.

Lottrup G et al. (2006). Possible impact of phthalates on infant reproductive health. *International Journal of Andrology*, 29:172–180.

Luczynska CM et al. (1989). A two-site monoclonal antibody ELISA for the quantification of the major *Dermatophagoides* spp. allergens, Der p I and Der f I. *Journal of Immunological Methods*, 118:227–235.

Luosujärvi RA et al. (2003). Joint symptoms and diseases associated with moisture damage in a health center. *Clinical Rheumatology*, 22:381–385.

Macher J, ed. (1999). *Bioaerosols: assessment and control*. Cincinnati, American Conference of Governmental Industrial Hygienists.

Macher JM, Huang FY, Flores M (1991). A two-year study of microbiological indoor air quality in a new apartment. *Archives of Environmental Health*, 46:25–29.

Madigan M, Martinko J, eds. (2005). *Brock biology of microorganisms*, 11th ed. Upper Saddle River, NJ, Prentice Hall.

Maier WC et al. (1997). Indoor risk factors for asthma and wheezing among Seattle school children. *Environmental Health Perspectives*, 105:208–214.

Malmberg P et al. (1985). Exposure to microorganisms, febrile and airway-obstructive symptoms, immune status and lung function of Swedish farmers. *Scandinavian Journal of Work, Environment and Health*, 11:287–293.

Martin TR, Frevert CW (2005). Innate immunity in the lungs. *Proceedings of the American Thoracic Society*, 2:403–411.

Marx JJ et al. (1990). Cohort studies of immunologic lung disease among Wisconsin dairy farmers. *American Journal of Industrial Medicine*, 18:263–268.

Mason CD et al. (2001). Effects of *Stachybotrys chartarum* on surfactant convertase activity in juvenile mice. *Toxicology and Applied Pharmacology*, 172:21–28.

Matheson MC et al. (2005). Changes in indoor allergen and fungal levels predict changes in asthma activity among young adults. *Clinical and Experimental Allergy*, 35:907–913.

Mattson J, Carlson OE, Engh IB (2002). Negative influence on IAQ by air movement from mould contaminated constructions into buildings. In: *Proceedings of Indoor Air 2002, 9th International Conference on Indoor Air Quality and Climate, Monterey, California, 30 June – 5 July 2002*. Vol.1. Atlanta, American Society of Heating Refrigerating and Air Conditioning Engineers:764–769.

Meklin T et al. (2007). Comparison of mold concentrations quantified by MSQPCR in indoor and outdoor air sampled simultaneously. *Science of the Total Environment*, 382:130–134.

Mendell MJ, Smith AH (1990). Consistent pattern of elevated symptoms in air-conditioned office buildings: a reanalysis of epidemiologic studies. *American Journal of Public Health*, 80:1193–1199.

Mendell MJ et al. (1996). Elevated symptom prevalence associated with ventilation type in office buildings. *Epidemiology*, 7:583–589.

Mendell MJ et al. (2003). Environmental risk factors and work-related lower respiratory symptoms in 80 office buildings: an exploratory analysis of NIOSH
data. *American Journal of Industrial Medicine*, 43:630–641.

Mendell MJ et al. (2006). Indicators of moisture and ventilation system contamination in US office buildings as risk factors for respiratory and mucous membrane symptoms: analyses of the EPA BASE data. *Journal of Occupational and
Environmental Hygiene*, 3:225–233.

Mendell MJ et al. (2007). *Risk factors in heating, ventilating, and air–conditioning
systems for occupant symptoms in US office buildings: the US EPA BASE Study.*
Berkeley, Lawrence Berkeley National Laboratory (Report LBNL-61870).

Mendell MJ et al. (2008). Risk factors in heating, ventilating, and air-conditioning systems for occupant symptoms in US office buildings: the US EPA BASE
study. *Indoor Air*, 18:301–316

Menzies D et al. (2000). Hospital ventilation and risk for tuberculous infection in
Canadian health care workers. Canadian Collaborative Group in Nosocomial
Transmission of TB. *Annals of Internal Medicine*, 133: 779–789.

Menzies D et al. (2003). Effect of ultraviolet germicidal lights installed in office
ventilation systems on workers' health and wellbeing: double-blind multiple
crossover trial. *Lancet*, 362:1785–1791.

Meyer HW et al. (2005). Double blind placebo controlled exposure to moulds:
exposure system and clinical results. *Indoor Air*, 15(Suppl. 10):73–80.

Meyer V, Stahl U (2003). The influence of co-cultivation on expression of the an-
tifungal protein in *Aspergillus giganteus*. *Journal of Basic Microbiology*, 43:68–
74.

Michel O et al. (1996). Severity of asthma is related to endotoxin in house dust.
American Journal of Respiratory and Critical Care Medicine, 154:1641–1646.

Milanowski J (1998). Effect of inhalation of organic dust-derived microbial
agents on the pulmonary phagocytic oxidative metabolism of guinea pigs.
Journal of Toxicology and Environmental Health A, 53:5–18.

Miller JD, Young JC (1997). The use of ergosterol to measure exposure to fungal propagules in indoor air. *American Industrial Hygiene Association Journal*,
58:39–43.

Ministry of Social Affairs and Health (2003). *Asumisterveysohje. Asuntojen ja
muiden oleskelutilojen fysikaaliset, kemialliset ja mikrobiologiset tekijät. Sos-
iaali- ja terveysministeriö. Oppaita 1. [Health Protection Act. Instructions regarding physical, chemical and biological factors in housing. Guidebook No. 1].*
Helsinki, Ministry of Social Affairs and Health (in Finnish).

Mohamed N et al. (1995). Home environment and asthma in Kenyan schoolchildren: a case-control study. *Thorax*, 50:74–78.

Mommers M et al. (2005). Indoor environment and respiratory symptoms in
children living in the Dutch–German borderland. *International Journal of Hygiene and Environmental Health*, 208:373–381.

Morrison DC, Ryan JL (1979). Bacterial endotoxins and host immune responses. *Advances in Immunology*, 28:293–434.

Morrison G, Hodgson A (1996). Evaluation of ventilation system materials as sources of volatile organic compounds. In: *Proceedings of the 7th International Conference of Indoor Air Quality and Climate*. Atlanta, American Society of Heating Refrigerating and Air Conditioning Engineers, 3:585–590.

Morrison G et al. (1998). Indoor air quality impacts of ventilation ducts: ozone removal and emissions of volatile organic compounds. *Journal of the Air and Waste Management Association*, 48:941–952.

Mosley RB et al. (2001). Penetration of ambient fine particles into the indoor environment. *Aerosol Science and Technology*, 34:127–136.

Moularat S, Robine E (2008). A method to determine the transfer of mycotoxins from materials to air. *CLEAN — Soil, Air, Water*, 36:578–583.

Moularat S et al. (2008a). Detection of fungal development in closed spaces through the determination of specific chemical targets. *Chemosphere*, 72:224–232.

Moularat S et al. (2008b). Detection of fungal development in a closed environment through the identification of specific VOC: demonstration of a specific VOC fingerprint for fungal development. *Science of the Total Environment*. 407:139-146.

Mudarri D, Fisk WJ (2007). Public health and economic impact of dampness and mold. *Indoor Air*, 17:226–235.

Mukhopadhyaya P et al. (2003). *Long-term performance: predict the moisture management performance of wall systems as a function of climate, material properties, etc. through mathematical modelling.* Ottawa, Institute for Research in Construction (Research Report IRC-RR-132):384.

Müller A et al. (2002). Increased incidence of allergic sensitisation and respiratory diseases due to mould exposure: results of the Leipzig Allergy Risk children Study (LARS). *International Journal of Hygiene and Environmental Health*, 204:363–365.

Murtoniemi T, Nevalainen A, Hirvonen MR (2003). Effect of plasterboard composition on *Stachybotrys chartarum* growth and biological activity of spores. *Applied and Environmental Microbiology*, 69:3751–3757.

Murtoniemi T et al. (2001a). Production of inflammatory mediators in RAW264.7 macrophages by microbes grown on six different plasterboards. *Inhalation Toxicology*, 13:233–247.

Murtoniemi T et al. (2001b). Induction of cytotoxicity and production of inflammatory mediators in RAW264.7 macrophages by spores grown on six different plasterboards. *Inhalation Toxicology*, 13:233–247.

Murtoniemi T et al. (2002). Effect of liner and core materials of plasterboard on microbial growth, spore-induced inflammatory responses, and cytotoxicity in macrophages. *Inhalation Toxicology*, 14:1087–1101.

Murtoniemi T et al. (2003). The relation between growth of four microbes on six different plasterboards and biological activity of spores. *Indoor Air*, 13:65–73.

Murtoniemi T et al. (2005). Effects of microbial cocultivation on inflammatory and cytotoxic potential of spores. *Inhalation Toxicology*, 17:681–693.

Myllykangas-Luosujärvi R et al. (2002). A cluster of inflammatory rheumatic diseases in a moisture-damaged office. *Clinical and Experimental Rheumatology*, 20:833–836.

Nafstad P et al. (1998). Residential dampness problems and symptoms and signs of bronchial obstruction in young Norwegian children. *American Journal of Respiratory and Critical Care Medicine*, 157:410–414.

Nafstad P et al. (2005). Day care center characteristics and children's respiratory health. *Indoor Air*, 15:69–75.

Nevalainen A et al. (1998). Prevalence of moisture problems in Finnish houses. *Indoor Air*, 4(Suppl.):45–49.

Nguyen Thi LC, Kerr G, Johanson J (2000) Monitoring and remediation after a flood in a Canadian office building. In: *Proceedings of Healthy Buildings 2000.* Vol.3. Espoo, Sisällmastoseminaarit:433–438.

Nicolai T, Illi S, von Mutius E (1998). Effect of dampness at home in childhood on bronchial hyperreactivity in adolescence. *Thorax*, 53:1035–1040.

Nielsen KF et al. (1999). Production of mycotoxins on artificially and naturally infested building materials. *Mycopathologia*, 145:43–56.

Nielsen KF et al. (2002). Metabolite profiles of *Stachybotrys* isolates from water-damaged buildings and their induction of inflammatory mediators and cytotoxicity in macrophages. *Mycopathologia*, 154:201–205.

Nikulin M et al. (1996). Experimental lung mycotoxicosis in mice induced by *Stachybotrys atra*. *International Journal of Experimental Pathology*, 77:213–218.

Nikulin M et al. (1997). Effects of intranasal exposure to spores of *Stachybotrys atra* in mice. *Fundamental and Applied Toxicology*, 35:182–188.

Norbäck D et al. (1999). Current asthma and biochemical signs of inflammation in relation to building dampness in dwellings. *International Journal of Tuberculosis and Lung Disease*, 3:368–376.

Norbäck D et al. (2000). Asthma symptoms in relation to measured building dampness in upper concrete floor construction, and 2-ethyl-1-hexanol in indoor air. *International Journal of Tuberculosis and Lung Disease*, 4:1016–1025.

Nordenbo AM, Gravesen S (1979). Allergisk alveolitis forårsaget af en kontamineret befugter [Allergic alveolitis caused by a contaminating humidifier]. *Ugeskrift for Læger*, 141:886–887 (in Dannish).

Nriagu J et al. (1999). Prevalence of asthma and respiratory symptoms in south-central Durban, South Africa. *European Journal of Epidemiology*, 15:747–755.

Øie L et al. (1999). Ventilation in homes and bronchial obstruction in young children. *Epidemiology*, 10:294–299.

Olsen JH, Dragsted L, Autrup H (1988). Cancer risk and occupational exposure to aflatoxins in Denmark. *British Journal of Cancer*, 58:392–396.

Osborne M et al. (2006). Specific fungal exposures, allergic sensitization, and rhinitis in infants. *Pediatric Allergy and Immunology*, 17:450–457.

Özkaynak H et al. (1996). Personal exposure to airborne particles and metals: results from the particle TEAM study in Riverside, California. *Journal of Exposure Analysis and Environmental Epidemiology*, 6:57–78.

Park JH et al. (2000). Longitudinal study of dust and airborne endotoxin in the home. *Environmental Health Perspectives*, 108:1023–1028.

Park JH et al. (2001). House dust endotoxin and wheeze in the first year of life. *American Journal of Respiratory and Critical Care Medicine*, 163:322–328.

Park JH et al. (2004). Building-related respiratory symptoms can be predicted with semi-quantitative indices of exposure to dampness and mold. *Indoor Air*, 14:425–433.

Park JH et al. (2006). Fungal and endotoxin measurements in dust associated with respiratory symptoms in a water-damaged office building. *Indoor Air*, 16:192–203.

Pasanen P ed. (2007). *Cleanliness of ventilation systems*. Brussels, Federation of European Heating and Air-conditioning Associations (Guidebook No.8).

Pasanen P et al. (2001). Fungal growth on wood surfaces at different moisture conditions in crawl spaces. In: *Moisture, microbes and health effects: indoor air quality and moisture in buildings. Proceedings of the International Building Performance Conference* [CD-ROM]. San Francisco, American Society of Heating, Refrigerating and Air-Conditioning Engineers.

Peat JK, Dickerson J, Li J (1998). Effects of damp and mould in the home on respiratory health: a review of the literature. *Allergy*, 53:120–128.

Pedersen B, Gravesen S (1983). Allergisk alveolitis på grund af mikroorganismer i indeklimaet [Allergic alveolitis precipitated by microorganisms in the home environment]. *Ugeskrift for Læger*, 145:580–581 (in Danish).

Pekkanen J et al. (2007). Moisture damage and childhood asthma: a population-based incident case-control study. *European Respiratory Journal*, 29:509–515.

Penttinen P et al. (2005a). The proportions of *Streptomyces californicus* and *Stachybotrys chartarum* in simultaneous exposure affect inflammatory responses in mouse RAW264.7 macrophages. *Inhalation Toxicology*, 17:79–85.

Penttinen P et al. (2005b). Interactions between *Streptomyces californicus* and *Stachybotrys chartarum* can induce apoptosis and cell cycle arrest in mouse RAW264.7 macrophages. *Toxicology and Applied Pharmacology*, 202:278–288.

Penttinen P et al. (2006). Co-cultivation of *Streptomyces californicus* and *Stachybotrys chartarum* stimulates the production of cytostatic compound(s) with immunotoxic properties. *Toxicology and Applied Pharmacology*, 217:342–351.

Penttinen P et al. (2007). DNA damage and p53 in RAW264.7 cells induced by the spores of co-cultivated *Streptomyces californicus* and *Stachybotrys chartarum*. *Toxicology*, 235:92–102.

Pessi AM et al. (2002). Microbial growth inside insulated external walls as an indoor air biocontamination source. *Applied and Environmental Microbiology*, 68:963–967.

Peters JM et al. (1999). A study of twelve Southern California communities with differing levels and types of air pollution. I. Prevalence of respiratory morbidity. *American Journal of Respiratory and Critical Care Medicine*, 159:760–767.

Pettigrew MM et al. (2004). Association of early-onset otitis media in infants and exposure to household mould. *Paediatric and Perinatal Epidemiology*, 18:441–447.

Phalen RF et al. (2006). Tracheobronchial particle dose concentrations for in vitro toxicology studies. *Toxicolocical Sciences*, 92:126–132.

Pieckova E, Jesenska Z (1996). Ciliostatic effect of fungi on the respiratory tract ciliary movement of one-day-old chickens in vitro. *Folia Microbiologica*, 41:517–520.

Pieckova E, Jesenska Z (1998). Molds on house walls and the effect of their chloroform-extractable metabolites on the respiratory cilia movement of one-day-old chicks in vitro. *Folia Microbiologica*, 43:672–678.

Pieckova E et al. (2006). Pulmonary cytotoxicity of secondary metabolites of *Stachybotrys chartarum* (Ehrenb.) Hughes. *Annals of Agricultural and Environmental Medicine*, 13:259–262.

Pirhonen I et al. (1996). Home dampness, moulds and their influence on respiratory infections and symptoms in adults in Finland. *European Respiratory Journal*, 9:2618–2622.

Pirinen J (2006). *Damages caused by microbes in small houses*. Tampere, Tampere University of Technology.

Pirinen J et al. (2005). *Homevauriot suomalaisissa pientaloissa [Mould damage in Finnish detached houses]*. Espoo, Sisäilmastoseminaari (SIY Report 23; in Finnish).

Pollart SM et al. (1994). Environmental exposure to cockroach allergens: analysis with monoclonal antibody-based enzyme immunoassays. *Journal of Allergy and Clinical Immunology*, 87:505–510.

Ponsonby AL et al. (2000). The relation between infant indoor environment and subsequent asthma. *Epidemiology*, 11:128–135.

Price JA et al. (1990). Measurement of airborne mite antigen in homes of asthmatic children. *Lancet*, 336:895–897.

Purokivi MK et al. (2001). Changes in pro-inflammatory cytokines in association with exposure to moisture-damaged building microbes. *European Respiratory Journal*, 18:951–958.

Pylkkänen L et al. (2004). Exposure to *Aspergillus fumigatus* spores induces chemokine expression in mouse macrophages. *Toxicology*, 200:255–263.

Rand TG et al. (2003). Histological, immunohistochemical and morphometric changes in lung tissue in juvenile mice experimentally exposed to *Stachybotrys chartarum* spores. *Mycopathologia*, 156:119–131.

Rand TG et al. (2006). Comparison of inflammatory responses in mouse lungs exposed to atranones A and C from *Stachybotrys chartarum*. *Journal of Toxicology and Environmental Health, Part A*, 69:1239–1251.

Rao CY, Brain JD, Burge HA (2000). Reduction of pulmonary toxicity of *Stachybotrys chartarum* spores by methanol extraction of mycotoxins. *Applied and Environmental Microbiology*, 66:2817–2821.

Rao CY, Burge HA, Brain JD (2000). The time course of responses to intratracheally instilled toxic *Stachybotrys chartarum* spores in rats. *Mycopathologia*, 149:27–34.

Rask-Andersen A (1988). *Pulmonary reactions to inhalation of mould dust in farmers with special reference to fever and allergic alveolitis* [thesis]. Uppsala, Universitatis Uppsaliensis.

Rask-Andersen A et al. (1994) Inhalation fever and respiratory symptoms in the trimming department of Swedish sawmills. *American Journal of Industrial Medicine*, 25:65–67.

REHVA (2007a). *Cleanliness of ventilation systems*. Brussels, Federation of European Heating and Air-conditioning Associations (Guidebook No. 8).

REHVA (2007b). *Hygiene requirement for ventilation and air-conditioning*. Brussels, Federation of European Heating and Air-conditioning Associations (Guidebook No. 9).

Reinikainen L, Jaakkola J (2003). Significance of humidity and temperature on skin and upper airway symptoms. *Indoor Air*, 13:344–352.

Rennie D et al. (2005). Differential effect of damp housing on respiratory health in women. *Journal of the American Medical Women's Association*, 60:46–51.

Reponen T (1995). Aerodynamic diameters and respiratory deposition estimated of viable particles in mold problem dwellings, *Aerosol Science and Technology*, 22:11–23.

Reynolds S et al. (2002). Interlaboratory comparison of endotoxin assays using agricultural dusts. *American Industrial Hygiene Association Journal*, 63:430–438.

Rietschel ET et al. (1985). Newer aspects of the chemical structure and biological activity of bacterial endotoxins. In: ten Cate J, Buller HW, ten Cate JW, eds. *Bacterial endotoxins: structure, biomedical significance, and detection with the Limulus amebocyte lysate test*. New York, Alan Liss: 31–50.

Riggi SJ, Di Luzio NR (1961). Identification of a reticuloendothelial stimulating agent in zymosan. *American Journal of Physiology*, 200:297–300.

Rintala H, Nevalainen A, Suutari M (2002). Diversity of streptomycetes in water-damaged building materials based on 16S rDNA sequences. *Letters in Applied Microbiology*, 34:439–443.

Rintala H et al. (2004). Detection of streptomycetes in house dust – comparison of culture and PCR methods. *Indoor Air*, 14:112–119.

Robine E et al. (2005). Characterisation of exposure to airborne fungi: measurement of ergosterol. *Journal of Microbiological Methods*, 63:185–192.

Rocha O, Ansari K, Doohan FM (2005). Effects of trichothecene mycotoxins on eukaryotic cells: a review. *Food Additives and Contaminants*, 22:369–378.

Ronald PT (1994). Relevant moisture properties of building construction materials. In: Trechsel HR, ed. *Moisture control in buildings*. Philadelphia, American Society for Testing and Materials (ASTM manual series, MNL 18).

Rönmark E et al. (1999). Different pattern of risk factors for atopic and nonatopic asthma among children – report from the Obstructive Lung Disease in Northern Sweden Study. *Allergy*, 54:926–935.

Roponen M et al. (2001). Differences in inflammatory responses and cytotoxicity in RAW264.7 macrophages induced by *Streptomyces anulatus* grown on different building materials. *Indoor Air*, 11:179–184.

Rosenblum Lichtenstein JH et al. (2006). Strain differences influence murine pulmonary responses to *Stachybotrys chartarum*. *American Journal of Respiratory Cell and Molecular Biology*, 35:415–423.

Rotter BA, Prelusky DB, Pestka JJ (1996). Toxicology of deoxynivalenol (vomitoxin). *Journal of Toxicology and Environmental Health*, 48:1–34.

Rowan NJ et al. (1999). Prediction of toxigenic fungal growth in buildings by using a novel modelling system. *Applied and Environmental Microbiology*, 65:4814–4821.

Roy CJ, Thorne PS (2003). Exposure to particulates, microorganisms, $\beta(1\text{-}3)$-glucans, and endotoxins during soybean harvesting. *American Industrial Hygiene Association Journal*, 64:487–495.

Ruotsalainen R, Jaakkola N, Jaakkola JJ (1995). Dampness and molds in day-care centers as an occupational health problem. *International Archives of Occupational and Environmental Health*, 66:369–374.

Rylander R (1994). The first case of sick building syndrome in Switzerland. *Indoor and Built Environment*, 3:159–162.

Rylander R (1996). Airway responsiveness and chest symptoms after inhalation of endotoxin or $(1\rightarrow3)\text{-}\beta\text{-}D$-glucan. *Indoor and Built Environment*, 5:106–111.

Rylander R (1997a). $(1\rightarrow3)\text{-}\beta\text{-}D$-glucan in some indoor air fungi. *Indoor and Built Environment*, 6:291–294.

Rylander R (1997b). Airborne $(1\rightarrow3)\text{-}\beta\text{-}D$-glucan and airway disease in a day-care center before and after renovation. *Archives of Environmental Health*, 52:281–285.

Rylander R (1999). Indoor air-related effects and airborne (1→3)-β-D-glucan. *Environmental Health Perspectives*, 107(Suppl. 3):501–503.

Rylander R, Fogelmark B (1994). Inflammatory responses by inhalation of endotoxin and (1→3)-β-D-glucan. *American Journal of Industrial Medicine*, 25:101–102.

Rylander R, Fogelmark B, Danielsson B (1998). Glukan i inomhusmiljö gav luftvägsinflammation [Did glucan in indoor environment cause respiratory tract inflammation]? *Läkartidningen*, 95:1562–1563 (in Swedish).

Rylander R, Holt PG (1998). (1→3)-β-D-Glucan and endotoxin modulate immune response to inhaled allergen. *Mediators of Inflammation*, 7:105–110.

Rylander R, Mégevand Y (2000). Environmental risk factors for respiratory infections. *Archives of Environmental Health*, 55:300–303.

Rylander R et al. (1989). The importance of endotoxin and glucan for symptoms in sick buildings. In: Bieva CJ et al., eds. *Present and future of indoor air quality*. Amsterdam, Excerpta Medica:219–226.

Rylander R et al. (1992). Airborne beta-1,3-glucan may be related to symptoms in sick buildings. *Indoor and Built Environment*, 1:263–267.

Rylander R et al. (1998). Airways inflammation, atopy, and (1→3)-β-D-glucan exposure in two schools. *American Journal of Respiratory and Critical Care Medicine*, 158:1685–1687.

Saijo Y et al. (2004). Symptoms in relation to chemicals and dampness in newly built dwellings. *International Archives of Occupational and Environmental Health*, 77:461–470.

Salo PM et al. (2006). Exposure to *Alternaria alternata* in US homes is associated with asthma symptoms. *Journal of Allergy and Clinical Immunology*, 118:892–898.

Salonvaara M, Nieminen J (2002). Hygrothermal performance of low-sloped roofs with groove ventilation. In: Gustavsen A, Thue, JV, eds. *Proceedings of the 6th Symposium on Building Physics in the Nordic Countries, 17–19 June, Trondheim*. Trondheim, Norwegian University of Science and Technology:239–246.

Samson RA et al., eds (1994). *Health implications of fungi in indoor environments*. New York, Elsevier.

Säteri J, Kovanen K, Pallari ML (1999). *Kerrostalojen sisäilmaston ja energiataalouden parantaminen [Improvements of indoor air quality and energy efficiency in hige-rise residential buildings]*. Espoo, VTT Technical Research Centre (VTT Research Notes 1945; in Finnish).

Schäfer T et al. (1999). What makes a child allergic? Analysis of risk factors for allergic sensitization in preschool children from East and West Germany. *Allergy and Asthma Procedeedings*, 20:23–27.

Schellen HL et al. (2004). Indoor air humidity of massive buildings and hygro-thermal surface conditions. In: *Proceedings of the 9th Conference on Performance of Exterior Envelopes of Whole Buildings, 5–10 December 2004, Clearwater Beach, Florida* [CD-ROM]. Atlanta, American Society of Heating Refrigerating and Air Conditioning Engineers.

Schou C, Svendsen UG, Lowenstein H (1991). Purification and characterization of the major dog allergen, Can f I. *Clinical and Experimental Immunology*, 21:321–328.

Schwarz H, Wettengel R, Kramer B (2000). Extrinsic allergic alveolitis in domestic environments (domestic allergic alveolitis) caused by mouldy tapestry. *European Journal of Medical Research*, 5:125.

Schwarze PE et al. (2007). Importance of size and composition of particles for effects on cells in vitro. *Inhalation Toxicology*, 19(Suppl. 1):17–22.

Sedlbauer K (2001). *Vorhersage von Schimmelpilzbildung auf und in Bauteilen* [thesis]. Stuttgart, University of Stuttgart.

Selim MI, Juchems AM, Popendorf W (1998). Assessing airborne aflatoxin B1 during on-farm grain handling activities. *American Industrial Hygiene Association Journal*, 59:252–256.

Seppänen O (2004). Improvement of indoor environment in European residences to alleviate the symptoms of allergic and asthmatic children and adults. In: Franchi et al., eds. *Towards healthy air in dwellings in Europe. The THADE report.* [CD-ROM]. Brussels, European Federation of Allergy and Airways Diseases Patient Associations.

Seppänen OA, Fisk WJ (2002). Association of ventilation system type with SBS symptoms in office workers. *Indoor Air*, 12:98–112.

Seppänen O, Fisk WJ (2004). Summary of human responses to ventilation. *Indoor Air*, 14(Suppl. 7):102–118.

Seppänen O, Fisk WJ, Lei QH (2006). Ventilation and performance in office work. *Indoor Air*, 16:28–36.

Seppänen O, Fisk W, Mendell M (1999). Association of ventilation rates and CO_2 concentrations with health and other responses in commercial and institutional buildings. *Indoor Air*, 9:226–252.

Seuri M et al. (2000). An outbreak of respiratory diseases among workers at a water-damaged building – a case report. *Indoor Air*, 10:138–145.

Shin SH et al. (2004) Chronic rhinosinusitis: an enhanced immune response to ubiquitous airborne fungi. *Journal of Allergy and Clinical Immunology*, 114:1369–1375.

Sieber WK et al. (1996). The National Institute for Occupational Safety and Health indoor environmental evaluation experience: part three – associations between environmental factors and self-reported health conditions. *Applied Occupational and Environmental Hygiene*, 11:1387–1392.

Siersted HC, Gravesen S (1993). Extrinsic allergic alveolitis after exposure to the yeast *Rhodotorula rubra*. *Allergy*, 48:298–299.

Sigsgaard T et al. (2000). Cytokine release from the nasal mucosa and whole blood after experimental exposures to organic dusts. *European Respiratory Journal*, 16:140–145.

Simoni M et al. (2005). Mould/dampness exposure at home is associated with respiratory disorders in Italian children and adolescents: the SIDRIA-2 Study. *Occupational and Environmental Medicine*, 62:616–622.

Simpson A et al. (2002). Household characteristics and mite allergen levels in Manchester, UK. *Clinical and Experimental Allergy*, 32:1413–1419.

Singh J (1999). Dry rot and other wood-destroying fungi: their occurrence, biology, pathology and control. *Indoor and Built Environment*, 8:3–20.

Sjöstrand M, Rylander R (1997). Pulmonary cell infiltration after chronic exposure to (1→3)-β-D-glucan and cigarette smoke. *Inflammation Research*, 46:93–97.

Skorge TD et al. (2005). Indoor exposures and respiratory symptoms in a Norwegian community sample. *Thorax*, 60:937–942.

Slezak JA et al. (1998). Asthma prevalence and risk factors in selected Head Start sites in Chicago. *Journal of Asthma*, 35:203–212.

Solomon GM et al. (2006). Airborne mold and endotoxin concentrations in New Orleans, Louisiana, after flooding, October through November 2005. *Environmental Health Perspectives*, 114:1381–1386.

Sonesson A et al. (1988). Determination of environmental levels of peptidoglycan and lipopolysaccharide using gas chromatography–mass spectrometry utilizing bacterial amino acids and hydroxy fatty acids as biomarkers. *Journal of Chromatography B*, 431:1–15.

Sonesson A et al. (1990). Comparison of the Limulus amebocyte lysate test and gas chromatography–mass spectrometry for measuring lipopolysaccharides (endotoxins) in airborne dust from poultry-processing industries. *Applied and Environmental Microbiology*, 56:1271–1278.

Sotir M, Yeatts K, Shy C (2003). Presence of asthma risk factors and environmental exposures related to upper respiratory infection-triggered wheezing in middle school-age children. *Environmental Health Perspectives*, 111:657–662.

Spengler JD et al. (2004). Housing characteristics and children's respiratory health in the Russian Federation. *American Journal of Public Health*, 94:657–662.

Stark HJ et al. (2005). The effects of *Aspergillus fumigatus* challenge on exhaled and nasal NO levels. *European Respiratory Journal*, 26:887–893.

Stark H et al. (2006). *Aspergillus fumigatus* challenge increases cytokine levels in nasal lavage fluid. *Inhalation Toxicology*, 18:1033–1039.

Stark PC et al. (2003). Fungal levels in the home and lower respiratory tract illnesses in the first year of life. *American Journal of Respiratory and Critical Care Medicine*, 168:232–237.

Stark PC et al. (2005). Fungal levels in the home and allergic rhinitis by 5 years of age. *Environmental Health Perspectives*, 113:1405–1409.

Stockmann-Juvala H et al. (2004). Oxidative stress induced by fumonisin B1 in continuous human and rodent neural cell cultures. *Free Radical Research*, 38:933–942.

Stockmann-Juvala H et al. (2006). Fumonisin B1-induced apoptosis in neuroblastoma, glioblastoma and hypothalamic cell lines. *Toxicology*, 225:234–241.

Stone BA, Clarke AE (1992). *Chemistry and biology of (1→3)-β-glucans*. Melbourne, Victoria, La Trobe University Press.

Strachan DP (1989). Hay fever, hygiene, and household size. *British Medical Journal*, 299:1259–1260.

Strachan DP (2000). Family size, infection and atopy: the first decade of the 'hygiene hypothesis'. *Thorax*, 55(Suppl. 1):S2–S10.

Strachan DP, Carey IM (1995). Home environment and severe asthma in adolescence: a population based case-control study. *British Medical Journal*, 311:1053–1056.

Strachan DP, Elton RA (1986). Relationship between respiratory morbidity in children and the home environment. *Family Practice*, 3:137–142.

Strachan DP et al. (1990). Quantification of airborne moulds in the homes of children with and without wheeze. *Thorax*, 45:382–387.

Sun Y, Sundell J, Zhang Y (2007). Validity of building characteristics and dorm dampness obtained in a self-administrated questionnaire. *Science of the Total Environment*, 387:276–282.

Sundell J, Levin H (2007). *Ventilation rates and health: report of an interdisciplinary review of the scientific literature. Final report*. Atlanta, American Society of Heating, Refrigerating and Air-conditioning Engineers.

Swanson MC, Agarwal MK, Reed CE (1985). An immunochemical approach to indoor aeroallergen quantitation with a new volumetric air sampler: studies with mice, roach, cat, mouse, and guinea pig antigens. *Journal of Allergy and Clinical Immunology*, 76:724–729.

Swingler GH (1990). Summer-type hypersensitivity pneumonitis in southern Africa. A report of 5 cases in one family. *South African Medical Journal*, 77:104–107.

Tanaka H (2004). Uncommon association of hypersensitivity pneumonitis by *Aspergillus* and pulmonary aspergilloma; a new clinical entity? *Internal Medicine*, 43:896–897.

Taskinen T et al. (1997). Moisture and mould problems in schools and respiratory manifestations in schoolchildren: clinical and skin test findings. *Acta Paediatrica*, 86:1181–1187.

Taskinen T et al. (1999). Asthma and respiratory infections in school children with special reference to moisture and mold problems in the school. *Acta Paediatrica*, 88:1373–1379.

Tavernier G et al. (2006). IPEADAM study: indoor endotoxin exposure, family status, and some housing characteristics in English children. *Journal of Allergy and Clinical Immunology*, 117:656–662.

Tham KW et al. (2007). Associations between home dampness and presence of molds with asthma and allergic symptoms among young children in the tropics. *Pediatric Allergy and Immunology*, 18:418–424.

Thorn J, Rylander R (1998). Airways inflammation and glucan in a rowhouse area. *American Journal of Respiratory and Critical Care Medicine*, 157:1798–1803.

Thorn J, Beijer L, Rylander R (1998). Airways inflammation and glucan exposure among household waste collectors. *American Journal of Industrial Medicine*, 33:463–470.

Thorn J, Brisman J, Toren K (2001). Adult-onset asthma is associated with self-reported mold or environmental tobacco smoke exposures in the home. *Allergy*, 56:287–292.

Thornburg J et al. (2001). Penetration of particles into buildings and associated physical factors. Part I: model development and computer simulations. *Aerosol Science and Technology*, 34:284–296.

Thorne PS et al. (1994). Bioaerosol sampling in field studies: Can samples be express mailed? *American Industrial Hygiene Association Journal*, 55:1072–1079.

Thorne PS et al. (1997). Field evaluation of endotoxin air sampling assay methods. *American Industrial Hygiene Association Journal*, 58:792–799.

Thorne PS et al. (2005). Endotoxin exposure is a risk factor for asthma: the national survey of endotoxin in United States housing. *American Journal of Respiratory and Critical Care Medicine*, 172:1371–1377.

Torok M, de Weck AL, Scherrer M (1981). Allergische Alveolitis infolge Verschimmelung der Schlafzimmerwand. *Schweizer Medizinische Wochenschrift*, 111:924–929.

Torvinen E et al. (2006). Mycobacteria and fungi in moisture-damaged building materials. *Applied and Environmental Microbiology*, 72:6822–6824.

Tuomainen A, Seuri M, Sieppi A (2004). Indoor air quality and health problems associated with damp floor coverings. *International Archives of Occupational and Environmental Health*, 77:222–226.

Turyk M et al. (2006). Environmental allergens and asthma morbidity in low-income children. *Journal of Asthma*, 43:453–457.

van Strien RT et al. (1994). Mite antigen in house dust: relationship with different housing characteristics in The Netherlands. *Clinical and Experimental Allergy*, 24:843–853.

van Strien RT et al. (2004). The influence of air conditioning, humidity, temperature and other household characteristics on mite allergen concentrations in the northeastern United States. *Allergy*, 59:645–652.

Venn AJ et al. (2003). Effects of volatile organic compounds, damp, and other environmental exposures in the home on wheezing illness in children. *Thorax*, 58:955–960.

Verein Deutscher Ingenieure (1997). *Hygienic standards for ventilation and air-conditioning systems – offices and assembly rooms*. Dusseldorf, Verein Deutscher Ingenieure (Association of German Engineers) (VDI 6022).

Verhoeff AP et al. (1994a). Fungal propagules in house dust. I. Comparison of analytic methods and their value as estimators of potential exposure. *Allergy*, 49:533–539.

Verhoeff AP et al. (1994b). Fungal propagules in house dust. II. Relation with residential characteristics and respiratory symptoms. *Allergy*, 49:540–547.

Verhoeff AP et al. (1995). Damp housing and childhood respiratory symptoms: the role of sensitization to dust mites and molds. *American Journal of Epidemiology*, 141:103–110.

Vesper SJ et al. (2005). Comparison of populations of mould species in homes in the UK and USA using mould-specific quantitative PCR. *Letters in Applied Microbiology*, 41:367–373.

Vesper S et al. (2007). Development of an environmental relative moldiness index for US homes. *Journal of Occupational and Environmental Medicine*, 49:829–833.

Vette AF et al. (2001). Characterization of indoor–outdoor aerosol concentration relationships during the Fresno PM exposure studies. *Aerosol Science and Technology*, 34:118–126.

Viana ME et al. (2002). An extract of *Stachybotrys chartarum* causes allergic asthma-like responses in a BALB/c mouse model. *Toxicological Sciences*, 70:98–109.

Viitanen H, Ritschkoff AC (1991). *Mould growth in pine and spruce sapwood in relation to air humidity and temperature*. Uppsala, Swedish University of Agricultural Sciences, Department of Forest Products (Report No. 221).

Viitanen H et al. (2000). Modelling mould growth and decay damages. In: *Proceedings of Healthy Buildings 2000*. Vol. 3. Espoo, Sisällmastoseminaarit:341–346.

von Assendelft A et al. (1979). Humidifier-associated extrinsic allergic alveolitis. *Scandinavian Journal of Work, Environment and Health*, 5:35–41.

von Mutius E (2007). Allergies, infections and the hygiene hypothesis — the epidemiological evidence. *Immunobiology*, 212:433–439.

Waegemaekers M et al. (1989). Respiratory symptoms in damp homes. A pilot study. *Allergy*, 44:192–198.

Wålinder R et al. (2001). Nasal lavage biomarkers: effects of water damage and microbial growth in an office building. *Archives of Environmental Health*, 56:30–36.

Walinder R et al. (2005). Acute effects of a fungal volatile compound. *Environmental Health Perspectives*, 113:1775–1778.

Wallace L (1996). Indoor particles: a review. *Journal of the Air and Waste Management Association*, 46:98–126.

Wan GH, Li CS (1999). Dampness and airway inflammation and systemic symptoms in office building workers. *Archives of Environmental Health*, 54:58–63.

Wan GH et al. (1999). An airbone mold-derived product, β-1,3-D-glucan, potentiates airway allergic responses. *European Journal of Immunology*, 29:2491–2497.

Wang H, Yadav JS (2006). DNA damage, redox changes, and associated stress-inducible signaling events underlying the apoptosis and cytotoxicity in murine alveolar macrophage cell line MH-S by methanol-extracted *Stachybotrys chartarum* toxins. *Toxicology and Applied Pharmacology*, 214:297–308.

Wargocki P, Wyon DP (2006a). The performance of school work by children is affected by classroom air quality and temperature. In: de Oliveira Fernandes E, Gameiro da Silva M, Rosado Pinto J, eds. *Creating a healthy indoor environment for people. Proceedings of Healthy Buildings 2006*. Rotterdam, International Council for Research and Innovation in Building and Construction:379.

Wargocki P, Wyon DP (2006b). Research report on effects of HVAC on student performance. *ASHRAE Journal*, 48:22–28.

Wargocki P, Wyon DP, Fanger PO (2004). The performance and subjective responses of call-center operators with new and used supply air filters at two outdoor air supply rates. *Indoor Air*, 14(Suppl. 8):7–16.

Wargocki W et al. (2002). Ventilation and health in non-industrial indoor environments. Report from a European multidisciplinary scientific consensus meeting. *Indoor Air*, 12:113–128.

Weschler C (2006). *Ozone's impact on public health: contributions from indoor exposures to ozone and products of ozone-initiated chemistry*. Research Triangle Park, National Institute of Environmental Health Sciences, National Institutes of Health, Department of Health and Human Services.

Wessén, B, Honkanen J, Mälarstig B (2002). Microorganisms, MVOCs and the health complaints. In: *Proceedings of Indoor Air 2002, 9th International Conference on Indoor Air Quality and Climate, Monterey, California*. Vol. 4. Atlanta, American Society of Heating Refrigerating and Air Conditioning Engineers:319–322.

Wever-Hess J et al. (2000). Risk factors for exacerbations and hospital admissions in asthma of early childhood. *Pediatric Pulmonology*, 29:250–256.

WHO Regional Office for Europe (2000a). *The right to healthy indoor air: report on a working group meeting, Bilthoven, The Netherlands, 15–17 May 2000*. Copenhagen, WHO Regional Office for Europe (http://www.euro.who.int/document/e69828.pdf, accessed 15 March 2009).

WHO Regional Office for Europe (2000b). *Air quality guidelines for Europe*, 2nd ed. Copenhagen, WHO Regional Office for Europe (European series No. 91; http://www.euro.who.int/document/e71922.pdf, accessed 16 March 2009).

WHO Regional Office for Europe (2006a). *Air quality guidelines global update 2005: particulate matter, ozone, nitrogen dioxide and sulfur dioxide*. Copenhagen, WHO Regional Office for Europe (http://www.euro.who.int/Document/E90038.pdf, accessed 14 June 2007).

WHO Regional Office for Europe (2006b). *Development of WHO guidelines for indoor air quality: report on a working group meeting, Bonn, Germany, 23–24 October 2006*. Copenhagen, WHO Regional Office for Europe (http://www.euro.who.int/Document/AIQ/IAQ_mtgrep_Bonn_Oct06.pdf, accessed 30 August 2007).

Wichmann G, Herbarth O, Lehmann I (2002). The mycotoxins citrinin, gliotoxin, and patulin affect interferon-gamma rather than interleukin-4 production in human blood cells. *Environmental Toxicology*, 17:211–218.

Wickens K et al. (1999). Indoor environment, atopy and the risk of asthma in children in New Zealand. *Pediatric Allergy and Immunology*, 10:199–208.

Wieslander G et al. (1999). Nasal and ocular symptoms, tear film stability and biomarkers in nasal lavage, in relation to building-dampness and building design in hospitals. *International Archives of Occupational and Environmental Health*, 72:451–461.

Wild LG, Lopez M (2001). Hypersensitivity pneumonitis: a comprehensive review. *Journal of Investigational Allergology and Clinical Immunology*, 11:3–15.

Wilkins K, Larsen K, Simkus M (2000). Volatile metabolites from mold growth on building materials and synthetic media. *Chemosphere*, 41:437–446.

Wilkins K, Larsen K, Simkus M (2003). Volatile metabolites from indoor molds grown on media containing wood constituents. *Environmental Science and Pollution Research International*, 10:206–208.

Williams DL (1997). Overview of (1→3)-β-D-glucan immunobiology. *Mediators of Inflammation*, 6:247–250.

Williamson IJ et al. (1997). Damp housing and asthma: a case-control study. *Thorax*, 52:229–234.

Wong GW et al. (2004). Factors associated with difference in prevalence of asthma in children from three cities in China: multicentre epidemiological survey. *British Medical Journal*, 329:486.

Wright RS et al. (1999). Hypersensitivity pneumonitis from *Pezizia domiciliana*: a case of El Niño lung. *American Journal of Respiratory and Critical Care Medicine*, 160:1758–1761.

Wucherpfennig KW (2001). Mechanisms for the induction of autoimmunity by infectious agents. *Journal of Clinical Investigation*, 108:1097–1104.

Wurtz H et al. (2005). The dustfall collector – a simple passive tool for long-term collection of airborne dust: a project under the Danish Mould in Buildings program (DAMIB). *Indoor Air*, 15(Suppl. 9):33–40.

Yang CY, Lin MC, Hwang KC (1998). Childhood asthma and the indoor environment in a subtropical area. *Chest*, 114:393–397.

Yang CY et al. (1997a). Damp housing conditions and respiratory symptoms in primary school children. *Pediatric Pulmonology*, 24:73–77.

Yang CY et al. (1997b). Effects of indoor environmental factors on respiratory health of children in a subtropical climate. *Environmental Research*, 75:49–55.

Yang CY et al. (1998). Indoor environmental risk factors and childhood asthma: a case-control study in a subtropical area. *Pediatric Pulmonology*, 26:120–124.

Yangzong et al. (2006). Childhood asthma under the north face of Mount Everest. *Journal of Asthma*, 43:393–398.

Yazicioglu M et al. (1998). Home environment and asthma in school children from the Edirne region in Turkey. *Allergologia et Immunopathologia (Madrid)*, 26:5–8.

Yike I, Rand TG, Dearborn DG (2005). Acute inflammatory responses to *Stachybotrys chartarum* in the lungs of infant rats: time course and possible mechanisms. *Toxicological Sciences*, 84:408–417.

Yike I, Rand T, Dearborn DG (2007). The role of fungal proteinases in pathophysiology of *Stachybotrys chartarum*. *Mycopathologia*, 164:171–181.

Yike I et al. (2002). Infant animal model of pulmonary mycotoxicosis induced by *Stachybotrys chartarum*. *Mycopathologia*, 154:139–152.

Yike I et al. (2006). Mycotoxin adducts on human serum albumin: biomarkers of exposure to *Stachybotrys chartarum*. *Environmental Health Perspectives*, 114:1221–1226.

Yli-Pirilä T et al. (2004). Amoebae and other protozoa in material samples from moisture-damaged buildings. *Environmental Research*, 96:250–256.

Yli-Pirilä T et al. (2007). Effects of co-culture of amoebae with indoor microbes on their cytotoxic and proinflammatory potential. *Environmental Toxicology*, 22:357–367.

Yoo CG et al. (1997) Summer-type hypersensitivity pneumonitis outside Japan: a case report and the state of the art. *Respirology*, 2:75–77 .

Zeng QY et al. (2006). Detection and quantification of *Cladosporium* in aerosols by real-time PCR. *Journal of Environmental Monitoring*, 8:153–160.

Zacharasiewicz A et al. (1999). Indoor factors and their association to respiratory symptoms suggestive of asthma in Austrian children aged 6–9 years. *Wiener Klinische Wochenschrift*, 111:882–886.

Zacharasiewicz A et al. (2000). Symptoms suggestive of atopic rhinitis in children aged 6–9 years and the indoor environment. *Allergy*, 55:945–950.

Zheng T et al. (2002). Childhood asthma in Beijing, China: a population-based case-control study. *American Journal of Epidemiology*, 156:977–983.

Zock JP et al. (2002). Housing characteristics, reported mold exposure, and asthma in the European Community Respiratory Health Survey. *Journal of Allergy and Clinical Immunology*, 110:285–292.

Zock JP et al. (2006). Distribution and determinants of house dust mite allergens in Europe: the European Community Respiratory Health Survey II. *Journal of Allergy and Clinical Immunology*, 118:682–690.

Zureik M et al. (2002). Sensitisation to airborne moulds and severity of asthma: cross sectional study from European Community respiratory health survey. *British Medical Journal*, 325:411–414.

Annex 1.
Summary of
epidemiological studies

Table A1.1. Epidemiological studies evaluated by the Institute of Medicine (2004), by category of health outcome associated with exposure to damp indoor environments or presence of mould or other agents in damp indoor environments

Reference	Participants

Asthma development

Adults
Population-based nested case-control studies

Jaakkola et al. (2002)	521 newly diagnosed adult cases; 932 controls
Thorn, Brisman, Toren (2001)	174 adults (aged 20–50 years) with asthma diagnosed in past 15 years 870 referents

Children
Nested and incident case-control studies

Øie et al. (1999)	172 children (aged < 2 years) with bronchial obstruction; 172 matched controls from population-based sample of 3754 newborns (same population as Nafstad et al., 1998)
Nafstad et al. (1998)	251 children (aged < 2 years) with bronchial obstruction 251 controls (aged 0–2 years) from population-based sample of 3754 newborns
Yang et al. (1998)	86 children with first diagnosis of asthma and 86 controls (aged 3–15 years)
Infante-Rivard (1993)	457 newly diagnosed cases and 457 controls (aged 3–4 years)

Cohort studies

Slezak et al. (1998)	1085 children in Head Start programmes (aged 3–5 years) with physician-diagnosed asthma
Maier et al. (1997)	925 children (aged 5–9 years) with current physician-diagnosed asthma followed prospectively for 1 year

Dampness or mould measure	Risk estimate (95% CI)
Visible mould or odour (work)	1.54 (1.01–2.32)
Damp stains or peeling paint (work)	0.84 (0.56–1.25)
Water damage (work)	0.91 (0.60–1.39)
Visible mould or odour (home)	0.98 (0.68–1.40)
Damp stains or peeling paint (home)	1.02 (0.73–1.41)
Water damage (home)	0.90 (0.61–1.34)
Self-reported visible dampness	1.3 (0.9–2.0)
Self-reported visible mould growth	2.2 (1.4–3.5)
Self-reported dampness or visible mould growth	1.8 (1.1–3.1) (prevalence)
Surveyor-verified dampness	2.4 (1.25–4.44)
Parent-reported dampness	2.5 (1.1–5.5)
Surveyor-verified dampness	3.8 (2.0–7.2)
Inspector-observed dampness	3.8 (2.0–7.2)
	Incidence of disease
Parent-reported dampness at home	1.77 (1.24–2.53)
Parent-reported humidifier use (not an indication of indoor dampness)	1.89 (1.30–2.74)
Self-reported dampness or mould	1.94 (1.23–3.04)
Water damage	1.7 (1.0–2.8)
Other wetness or no water damage	1.1 (0.6–1.8)

Reference	Participants

Upper respiratory tract symptoms

Adults
Cross-sectional studies

Engvall, Norrby, Norback (2002)	3241 adults living in multi-family buildings
Kilpeläinen et al. (2001)	10 667 students (aged 18–25 years)
Wan, Li (1999)	1113 workers in 19 office buildings
Wieslander et al. (1999)	95 staff members in four hospitals
Koskinen et al. (1999a)	699 adults (aged ≥ 16 years) in 310 households
Thorn, Rylander (1998)	129 adults (aged 18–83 years)
Pirhonen et al. (1996)	1460 adults (aged 25–64 years)
Brunekreef (1992)	2685 parents of children aged 6–12 years

Children
Cross-sectional studies

Rylander, Mégevand (2000)	304 children (aged 4–5 years)

Dampness or mould measure	Risk estimate (95% CI)
Self-reported mouldy odour and water leakage in past 5 years	1.92 (1.78–2.07) for nasal symptoms 4.42 (4.09–4.77) for throat irritation
Self-reported visible mould	1.29 (1.01–1.66) for allergic rhinitis 1.48 (1.17–1.88) for common cold ≥ 4 times per year
Self-reported visible mould, damp stains or water damage	1.30 (1.12–1.51) for allergic rhinitis 1.28 (1.09–1.47) for common cold ≥ 4 times per year
Self-reported mould	0.94 (0.50–1.77) for nasal congestion or runny nose
Self-reported flooding	1.55 (0.79–3.06) for nasal congestion or runny nose
Measured dampness in concrete floor	1.10 (1.02–1.18) for irritated, stuffy or runny nose
Surveyor-assessed moisture	1.06 (0.71–1.59) for rhinitis 1.92 (1.11–3.30) for sinusitis 1.46 (1.03–2.08) for sore throat
Self-reported mould	1.89 (1.15–3.11) for rhinitis 1.36 (0.78–2.39) for sinusitis 2.40 (1.56–3.69) for sore throat
Measured airborne glucans (> 2–4 ng/m^3)	1.23 (0.85–1.77) for nasal irritation
Self-reported dampness or mould problem	1.68 (0.97–2.89) for dry or sore throat
Self-reported damp stains or mould growth in past 2 years	1.03 (0.79–1.35) for allergy (women) 1.24 (0.95–1.73) for allergy (men)
Self-reported humidity	2.71 (1.07–6.91) for cold 3.02 (1.14–7.98) for sore throat
Self-reported mould at home	2.27 (0.082–6.33) for cold 2.57 (0.86–7.71) for sore throat

Reference	Participants
Zacharasiewicz et al. (2000)	2849 children (aged 6–9 years)
Dales, Miller (1999)	403 elementary-school children
Koskinen et al. (1999b)	204 children (aged ≤ 15 years) in 310 households
Jaakkola, Jaakkola, Ruotsalainen (1993)	2568 preschool children
Brunekreef et al. (1989)	4625 children (aged 7–11 years)

Cough

Adults
Cross-sectional studies

Reference	Participants
Gunnbjörnsdottir et al. (2003)	1853 young adults
Engvall, Norrby, Norbäck (2001)	3241 adults living in multifamily buildings
Koskinen et al. (1999a)	699 adults (aged ≥ 16 years) in 310 households
Thorn, Rylander (1998)	129 adults (aged 18–83 years)
Pirhonen et al. (1996)	1460 adults (aged 25–64 years)
Brunekreef (1992)	2685 parents of children aged 6–12 years

Dampness or mould measure	Risk estimate (95% CI)
Self-reported dampness at home	1.51 (1.31–1.74) for nasal symptoms
Self-reported mould or mildew	1.81 (1.02–3.24) for itchy eyes, skin rash or itch, nose irritation
Surveyor-assessed moisture	4.31 (1.80–10.34) for rhinitis 0.75 (0.19–2.98) for sinusitis 2.34 (1.13–4.86) for sore throat
Self-reported mould odour in past year	2.39 (1.15–4.98) for nasal congestion 2.38 (1.13–4.99) for nasal excretion
Self-reported water damage > 1 year ago	4.60 (2.57–8.22) for nasal congestion 3.19 (1.64–6.190) for nasal excretion
Self-reported mould (ever) Self-reported dampness (ever)	1.57 (1.31–1.87) for hay fever 1.26 (1.06–1.50) for hay fever

Self-reported water damage or visible mould at home ($n = 74$)	2.23 (1.24–4.00) for long-term cough
Self-reported mouldy odour and signs of high humidity Self-reported mouldy odour and major water leakage	3.97 (3.74–4.22) 3.78 (3.46–4.12)
Surveyor-assessed moisture	2.11 (1.21–4.98) for nocturnal cough 1.42 (0.92–2.19) for cough without phlegm 1.15 (0.78–1.69) for cough with phlegm
Self-reported mould	2.30 (1.32–4.01) for nocturnal cough 1.60 (1.01–2.53) for cough without phlegm 1.44 (0.95–2.19) for cough with phlegm
Measured airborne glucans (2–4 ng/m^3) Measured airborne glucans (> 4 ng/m^3)	1.05 (0.72–1.52) for dry cough 1.08 (0.74–1.56) for dry cough
Self-reported dampness or mould problem	1.37 (0.99–1.88)
Self-reported damp stains or mould growth (in past 2 years)	1.75 (1.30–2.36) among women 2.56 (1.94–3.38) among men

TABLE A1.1. CONT.

Reference	Participants
Waegemaekers et al. (1989)	164 adult men 164 adult women 190 children

Children
Cross-sectional studies

Reference	Participants
Belanger et al. (2003)	593 infants with sibling with asthma
	256 infants with sibling and mother with asthma
Gent et al. (2002)	880 infants (aged 1–12 months) with siblings with asthma
Dales, Miller (1999)	403 elementary-school children
Koskinen et al. (1999b)	204 children (aged ≤ 15 years) in 310 households
Taskinen et al. (1999)	622 children (aged 7–13 years); 101 cases
Andriessen, Brunekreef, Roemer (1998)	1614 children (aged 5–13 years)
Jędrychowski, Flak (1998)	1129 children (aged 9 years)
Rylander, Fogelmark, Danielsson (1998)	347 children at two schools (one with previous mould problem)

Dampness or mould measure	Risk estimate (95% CI)
Self-reported dampness at home	1.35 (NS; no CI reported)
Self-reported dampness at home	3.48 (NS; no CI reported)
Self-reported dampness at home	2.99 (1.28–6.97) for morning cough
	1.54 (0.77–3.10) for day
	or night cough
Author-measured airborne fungi	1.98 (no CI reported)
Reported persistent mould or mildew in previous 12 months	1.53 (1.01–2.30) for persistent cough
Measured fungal colonies (species not specified)	0.99 (0.89–1.10) for persistent cough
Reported persistent mould or mildew in previous 12 months	1.91 (1.07–3.42) for persistent cough
Measured fungal colonies (species not specified)	1.04 (0.87–1.24) for persistent cough
Measured *Penicillium* low (1–499 CFU/m^3)	1.01 (0.80–1.28)
Measured *Penicillium* medium (500–999 CFU/m^3)	1.62 (0.93–2.82)
Measured *Penicillium* high (≥ 1000 CFU/m^3)	2.06 (1.31–3.24)
Measured *Cladosporium* low (1–499 CFU/m^3)	1.03 (0.79–1.35)
Measured *Cladosporium* medium (500–999 CFU/m^3)	1.45 (0.99–2.12)
Measured *Cladosporium* high (≥ 1000 CFU/m^3)	0.72 (0.42–1.24)
"Other mould": low (1–499 CFU/m^3)	1.05 (0.83–1.33)
"Other mould": medium (500–999 CFU/m^3)	0.78 (0.42–1.45)
"Other mould": high (≥ 1000 CFU/m^3)	1.18 (0.63–2.21)
Water leaks	1.17 (0.91–1.49)
Humidifier use	1.26 (1.01–1.56)
Self-reported mould or mildew	1.28 (0.74–2.23) for nocturnal cough
	or wheeze
Surveyor-assessed moisture	5.72 (1.22–26.83) for nocturnal cough
	3.23 (1.43–7.31) for cough
	without phlegm
	0.94 (0.47–1.87) for cough
	with phlegm
Self-reported dampness (school)	2.3 (1.3–4.1)
Self-reported dampness (school and home)	4.7 (2.1–10.8)
Self-reported moisture stains	1.01 (0.89–1.16)
Self-reported mould	1.01 (0.87–1.18)
Self-reported mould or dampness	1.13 (0.64–2.02)
Problem school *vs* control school	26.1% *vs* 10.3% ($p = 0.024$) for
	nonatopic children (for dry cough)
	54.5% *vs* 7.1% ($p = 0.003$) for atopic
	children (for dry cough)

▶

Reference	Participants
Austin, Russell (1997)	1537 children (aged 12–14 years)
Jaakkola, Jaakkola, Ruotsalainen (1993)	2568 preschool children
Dales, Burnett, Zwanenburg (1991)	13 495 children (aged 5–8 years)
Dijkstra et al. (1990)	775 children (aged 6–12 years)
Brunekreef et al. (1989)	4625 children (aged 7–11 years)
Case-control studies	
Verhoeff et al. (1995)	Children (aged 6–12 years); 84 cases of chronic cough; 247 controls

Wheeze

Adolescents and adults
Cross-sectional studies

Gunnbjörnsdottir et al. (2003)	1853 young adults
Zock et al. (2002)	18 872 adults in 38 centres of the ECRHS

Dampness or mould measure	Risk estimate (95% CI)
	23.1% *vs* 8.2% ($p = 0.012$) for nonatopic children (for dry cough at night without cold)
	58.3% *vs* 6.5% ($p < 0.001$) for atopic children (for dry cough at night without cold)
	17.0% *vs* 7.5% (NS) for nonatopic children (for cough with phlegm)
	40.0% *vs* 7.1% ($p = 0.031$) for atopic children (for cough with phlegm)
Self-reported dampness	1.62 (1.06–2.48)
Self-reported mould	1.78 (1.10–2.89)
Self-reported mould odour in past year	3.88 (1.88–8.01) for persistent cough
Self-reported water damage > 1 year ago	2.54 (1.16–5.57) for persistent cough
Self-reported dampness or mould	1.89 (1.63–2.20)
Self-reported flooding	1.38 (1.16–1.65)
Self-reported moisture	1.91 (1.60–2.27)
Self-reported mould site	1.61 (1.36-1.89)
Self-reported mould sites (2 *vs* 0)	2.26 (1.80–2.83)
Self-reported damp stains or mould	0.57 (0.13–2.56)
Self-reported damp stains and mould	3.62 (1.57–8.36)
Self-reported mould (ever)	2.12 (1.64–2.73)
Self-reported dampness (ever)	2.16 (1.64–2.84)
Self-reported dampness	1.70 (0.94–3.09)
Self-reported mould	1.90 (1.02–3.52)
Surveyor-observed dampness	1.18 (0.70–1.99)
Surveyor-observed mould	1.26 (0.70–2.25)
Self-reported water damage or visible mould in home	1.4 (0.78–2.52)
Self-reported water damage in past year	1.16 (1.00–1.34) for wheeze and breathlessness
	1.23 (1.06–1.44) for wheeze (apart from colds)

▶

TABLE A1.1. CONT.

Reference	Participants
Nicolai, Illi, von Mutius (1998)	155 adolescents (mean age 13.5 years)
Brunekreef (1992)	2685 parents of children aged 6–12 years
Waegemaekers et al. (1989)	164 men 164 women 190 children
Case-control studies	
Norbäck et al. (1999)	98 cases and 357 controls nested in cohort of adults (aged 20–45 years)

Infants and children
Cross-sectional studies

Belanger et al. (2003) (same population as that studied by Gent et al., (2002))	849 infants with siblings with asthma
Gent et al. (2002)	880 infants (aged 1–12 months) with siblings with asthma

Dampness or mould measure	Risk estimate (95% CI)
Self-reported water on basement floor	1.46 (1.07–2.01) for wheeze and breathlessness 1.26 (0.81–1.98) for wheeze, (apart from colds)
Self-reported mould or mildew in last year	1.34 (1.18–1.51) for wheeze and breathlessness 1.44 (1.30–1.60) for wheeze, (apart from colds)
Self-reported dampness	14.3% exposed *vs* 5.3% ($p = 0.06$)
Self-reported dampness (adjusted for mite allergen levels)	5.77 (1.17–28.44)
Self-reported damp stains or mould growth (in past 2 years)	1.43 (1.15–1.77) in women 1.63 (1.30–2.06) in men
Self-reported damp at home	4.06 ($p < 0.01$; no CI reported)
Self-reported damp at home	4.79 ($p < 0.01$; no CI reported)
Self-reported damp at home	2.80 (1.18–6.64)
Author-measured airborne fungi	1.28 (includes shortness of breath and asthma)
Self-reported water damage or flooding	1.6 (1.03–2.6)
Dampness in the floor	2.8 (1.4–5.5)
Visible mould on indoor surfaces	2.4 (1.4–4.3)
Mouldy odour	1.5 (0.74–3.1)
At least one sign of dampness	2.2 (1.5–3.2)
Reported persistent mould or mildew in previous 12 months	2.51 (1.37–4.62) mother has asthma 1.22 (0.80–1.88) mother without asthma
Measured fungal colonies (species not specified)	1.23 (1.01–1.49) mother has asthma 1.10 (0.99–1.23) mother without asthma
Measured *Penicillium*: low (1–499 CFU/m^3)	1.11 (0.87–1.42)
Measured *Penicillium*: medium (500–999 CFU/m^3)	1.29 (0.65–1.48)
Measured *Penicillium*: high (≥ 1000 CFU/m^3)	2.15 (1.34–3.46)
Measured *Cladosporium*: low (1–499 CFU/m^3)	0.92 (0.69–1.22)
Measured *Cladosporium*: medium (500–999 CFU/m^3)	0.95 (0.61–1.49)
Measured *Cladosporium*: high (≥ 1000 CFU/m^3)	0.91 (0.53–1.56)
"Other mould": low (1–499 CFU/m^3)	0.97 (0.75–1.26)
"Other mould": medium (500–999 CFU/m^3)	0.91 (0.49–1.68)
"Other mould": high (≥ 1000 CFU/m^3)	1.02 (0.49–2.11)
Water leaks	1.18 (0.90–1.55)
Humidifier use	1.41 (1.11–1.79)

TABLE A1.1. CONT.

Reference	Participants
Park et al. (2001)	499 infants with at least one parent with asthma or allergy
Taskinen et al. (1999)	622 children (aged 7–13 years); 76 cases
Jędrychowski, Flak (1998)	1129 children (aged 9 years)
Rylander et al. (1998)	347 children in two schools (one with previous mould problem)
Slezak et al. (1998)	1085 children in Head Start programmes (aged 3–5 years)
Maier et al. (1997)	925 children (aged 5–9 years)
Jaakkola, Jaakkola, Ruotsalainen (1993)	2568 preschool children
Dales, Burnett, Zwanenburg (1991)	13 495 children (aged 5–8 years)
Dijkstra et al. (1990)	775 children (aged 6–12 years)
Strachan et al. (1990)	1000 children (aged 7 years)
Brunekreef et al. (1989)	4625 children (aged 7–11 years)

Dampness or mould measure	Risk estimate (95% CI)
Family room dust endotoxin level ≥ 100 units/mg	1.33 (0.99–1.79) for any wheeze 1.55 (1.00–2.42) for repeated wheeze
Self-reported dampness (school) Self-reported dampness (home) Self-reported dampness (school and home)	3.8 (1.8–8.3) 3.4 (0.8–14.2) 3.8 (1.3–11.3)
Self-reported mould or dampness	1.63 (1.07–2.48)

Problem school *vs* control school	13.5% *vs* 2.8% ($p = 0.014$)
	   for nonatopic children
	36.4% *vs* 13.3% (NS)
	   for atopic children

Self-reported dampness or mould	2.01 (1.38–2.93)
Self-reported mould Self-reported water damage Self-reported basement water Self-reported water condensation Any of the above	1.2 (0.7–1.9) 1.7 (1.0–2.8) 1.0 (0.6–1.7) 1.3 (0.8–2.1) 1.1 (0.7–1.8)
Self-reported mould odour in past year	4.31 (1.61–11.6) for persistent wheeze
Self-reported water damage > 1 year ago	8.67 (3.87–19.4) for persistent wheeze
Self-reported dampness or mould Self-reported flooding Self-reported moisture Self-reported mould site Self-reported mould sites (2 *vs* 0)	1.58 (1.42–1.76) 1.25 (1.10–1.41) 1.74 (1.53–1.98) 1.42 (1.26–1.59) 1.73 (1.45–2.06)
Self-reported damp stains or mould Self-reported damp stains and mould	1.13 (0.45–2.88) 1.54 (0.59–4.00)
Self-reported mould	3.70 (2.22–6.15)
Self-reported mould (ever) Self-reported dampness (ever)	1.79 (1.44–2.32) 1.23 (1.10–1.39)

Reference	Participants

Dyspnoea

Adults
Cross-sectional studies

Koskinen et al. (1999a)	699 adults (aged ≥ 16 years) in 310 households
Norbäck et al. (1999)	98 cases and 357 controls nested in a cohort of adults (aged 20–45 years)
Waegemaekers et al. (1989)	164 men 164 women 190 children

Children
Cross-sectional studies

Jędrychowski, Flak (1998)	1129 children (aged 9 years)

Asthma symptoms in people with asthma

Adults
Cross-sectional studies

Zock et al. (2002)	18 872 adults in 38 centres of the ECRHS
Kilpeläinen et al. (2001)	10 667 college students (aged 18–25 years)
Engvall, Norrby, Norbäck (2001)	3241 persons randomly sampled in multifamily buildings

Dampness or mould measure	Risk estimate (95% CI)
Surveyor-assessed moisture	2.33 (1.09–4.98) for nocturnal dyspnoea
Self-reported mould	1.58 (0.74–3.39) for nocturnal dyspnoea
Self-reported water damage or flooding	2.2 (1.4–3.7) daytime 2.2 (1.4–3.5) nocturnal
Dampness in the floor	3.1 (1.5–6.2) daytime 2.7 (1.3–5.4) nocturnal
Visible mould on indoor surfaces	2.2 (1.2–4.0) daytime 2.5 (1.4–4.5) nocturnal
Self-reported damp at home Self-reported damp at home Self-reported damp at home	9.38 (NS; no CI reported) 2.25 (NS; no CI reported) 0.92 (0.32–2.61)
Self-reported mould or dampness	2.01 (1.24–3.28)
Self-reported water damage in past year Self-reported water on basement floor Self-reported mould or mildew in past year	1.13 (0.95–1.35) for current asthma 1.54 (0.84–2.82) for current asthma 1.28 (1.13–1.46) for current asthma
Self-reported visible mould	2.21 (1.48–3.28) for current asthma symptoms
Self-reported visible mould, damp stains or water damage	1.66 (1.25–2.19) for current asthma symptoms
At least one sign of dampness	2.28 (2.19–2.37) for asthma symptoms

▶

Reference	Participants
Hu et al. (1997)	2041 young adults (aged 20–22 years)
Pirhonen et al. (1996)	1460 adults (aged 25–64 years)
Brunekreef (1992)	2685 parents of children aged 6–12 years
Waegemaekers et al. (1989)	164 men 164 women
Case-control studies	
Norbäck et al. (1999)	98 cases and 357 controls nested in a cohort of adults (aged 20–45 years)
Williamson et al. (1997)	102 people with asthma and 196 matched controls (aged 5–44 years)

Dampness or mould measure	Risk estimate (95% CI)
At least one dampness-related odour	2.38 (2.30–2.47) for asthma symptoms
Reports of at least one odour and structural building dampness	3.59 (3.37–3.82) for asthma symptoms
Self-reported water leak	1.6 (0.7–3.5) physician-reported 1.6 (0.7–3.8) self-reported
Self-reported indoor dampness	1.2 (0.8–1.9) physician-reported 1.3 (0.7–2.2) self-reported
Self-reported visible mould	1.5 (1.0–2.4) physician-reported 2.0 (1.2–3.2) self-reported
Self-reported damp or mould problem	1.02 (0.60–1.72)
Self-reported damps stains or mould growth (in past 2 years)	1.25 (0.94–1.66) among women 1.29 (0.92–1.81) among men
Self-reported damp at home Self-reported damp at home	1.15 (NS) 4.16 ($p < 0.05$)
Self-reported water damage or flooding	1.9 (1.2–2.9) for at least one asthma symptom
Dampness in the floor	3.3 (1.6–6.8) for at least one asthma symptom
Visible mould on indoor surfaces	2.9 (1.6–5.3) for at least one asthma symptom
Mouldy odour	1.8 (0.9–3.8) for at least one asthma symptom
At least one sign of dampness	2.2 (1.5–3.2) for at least one asthma symptom
Self-reported dampness or condensation in present dwelling	1.93 (1.14–3.28) physician-diagnosed asthma
Self-reported dampness in previous dwelling	2.55 (1.49–4.37) physician-diagnosed asthma
Observed severe dampness	2.36 (1.34–4.01) physician-diagnosed asthma
Observed significant mould	1.70 (0.78–3.71)

Reference	Participants
Children *Cross-sectional studies*	
Wever-Hess et al. (2000)	113 infants (aged 0–1 years)
Taskinen et al. (1999)	622 children (aged 7–13 years); 28 cases
Jędrychowski, Flak (1998)	1129 children (aged 9 years)
Nicolai, Illi, von Mutius (1998)	155 adolescents (mean age 13.5 years)
Rönmark et al. (1999)	3431 children (aged 7–8 years)
Yang et al. (1997a)	4164 primary-school children (aged 3–15 years)
Jaakkola, Jaakkola, Ruotsalainen (1993)	2568 preschool children
Dales, Burnett, Zwanenburg (1991)	13 495 children (aged 5–8 years)
Dijkstra et al. (1990)	775 children (aged 6–12 years)
Brunekreef et al. (1989)	4625 children (aged 7–11 years)
Waegemaekers et al. (1989)	190 children
Case-control studies	
Yazicioglu et al. (1998)	Children: 597 controls, 85 with asthma
Dekker et al. (1991)	13 495 children (aged 5–8 years)
Mohamed et al. (1995)	77 children with asthma and 77 controls (aged 9–11 years)

Source: Institute of Medicine (2004).

Dampness or mould measure	Risk estimate (95% CI)
Self-reported damp housing	7.6 (2.0–28.6) 3.8 (1.1–12.8) for recurrent exacerbation
Self-reported dampness (school)	1.0 (0.4–2.3) for symptomatic asthma
Self-reported dampness (home)	1.9 (0.4–10.4) for symptomatic asthma
Self-reported dampness (school and home)	1.1 (0.2–5.5) for symptomatic asthma
Self-reported mould or dampness	2.65 (0.96–7.13) for diagnosed asthma
Past or present self-reported dampness at home	61.5% exposed vs 37.7% unexposed (p < 0.05) for ≥ 5 asthma attacks in previous year
Parent-reported dampness at home	1.40 (0.81–2.42) for atopic asthma 1.78 (1.10–2.89) for nonatopic asthma
Self-reported dampness at home	1.73 (1.20–2.49) physician-confirmed asthma
Self-reported water damage > 1 year ago Self-reported mould odour in the past year	2.52 (0.93–6.87) 1.46 (0.34–6.29)
Self-reported flooding Self–reported moisture Self-reported dampness or mould Self-reported mould site Self-reported mould sites (2 vs 0)	1.29 (1.06–1.56) 1.58 (1.29–1.94) 1.45 (1.23–1.71) 1.40 (1.16–1.68) 1.67 (1.27–2.19)
Self-reported damp stains or mould Self-reported damp stains and mould	1.16 (0.38–3.52) 1.56 (0.50–4.87)
Self-reported dampness (ever)	1.42 (1.04–1.94)
Self-reported damp at home	2.80 (0.39–20.02)
Self-reported dampness at home	2.62 (1.13–6.81)
Self-reported dampness or visible mould	1.46 (1.22–1.74)
Author-observed damage from dampness in child's bedroom	4.9 (2.0–11.7)

Table A1.2. Articles not included in Institute of Medicine (2004) review on associations between health outcomes and dampness, mould or agents associated with dampness

Reference	Participants	Outcome

Asthma development

Adults
Prospective studies

Matheson et al. (2005)	845 adults (aged 20–45 years)	Doctor-diagnosed asthma

Retrospective studies

Gunnbjörnsdottir et al. (2006)	15 995 adults (aged 20–44 years) who participated in the ECRHS	Asthma onset

Children
Retrospective studies

Pekkanen et al. (2007)	362 children (aged 12–84 months) with asthma	New asthma diagnosis

Prospective studies

Jaakkola, Hwang, Jaakkola (2005)	1916 children (aged 1–7 years)	Asthma development

Dampness or mould measure	Risk estimate (95% CI)
Ergosterol[a]	1.50 (0.68–3.30)
Total fungi[a]	0.89 (0.60–1.34)
Other fungi[a]	0.99 (0.73–1.36
Cladosporium[a]	0.96 (0.72–1.27)
Dampness at home	1.13 (0.92–1.40)
Any suspected moisture damage at home	0.63 (0.28–1.45)
Area of water damage at home	1.01 (0.98–1.05)
Visible mould at home	1.24 (0.73–2.11)
Some mould odour at home	1.35 (0.42–4.36)
Clear mould odour at home	4.12 (0.65–26.01)
Minor or major moisture damage: main living area	2.24 (1.25–4.01)
Minor moisture damage: main living area	2.11 (1.06–4.21)
Major moisture damage: main living area	2.46 (1.09–5.55)
Maximum severity (1–2) moisture damage: main living area	2.75 (1.40–5.40)
Maximum severity (≥ 2) moisture damage: main living area	4.04 (1.60–10.20)
Area of damage in m^2	1.36 (0.91–2.03)
Mould growth, mould spots: main living area	4.01 (1.12–14.32)
Mould growth, visible mould: main living area	1.95 (0.69–5.47)
Visible mould: main living area	2.59 (1.15–5.85)
Mould odour: main living area	2.96 (0.62–14.19)
Minor or major moisture damage: kitchen	1.41 (0.80–2.47)
Visible mould: kitchen	1.13 (0.63–2.04)
Minor or major moisture damage: bathroom	0.70 (0.39–1.25)
Visible mould: bathroom	0.81 (0.44–1.49)
Minor or major moisture damage: other interior spaces	0.77 (0.40–1.46)
Visible mould: other interior spaces	0.86 (0.37–2.00)
Moisture damage: child's bedroom	1.97 (1.00–3.90)
Mould odour	IRR = 2.44 (1.07–5.60)
Visible mould	IRR = 0.65 (0.24–1.72)
Moisture on surfaces	IRR = 0.92 (0.54–1.54)
Water damage	IRR = 1.01 (0.45–2.26)

Reference	Participants	Outcome

Respiratory infections and otitis media

Adults
Cross-sectional studies

| Bakke et al. (2007) | 173 university staff in four university buildings | Airway infection last month |

Children
Prospective studies

Biagini et al. (2006)	663 infants enrolled in the Cincinnati Childhood Allergen and Air Pollution Study as of January 2004 with at least one parent with a positive skin-prick test	Upper respiratory infection in first year after birth
Pettigrew et al. (2004)	806 infants at high risk of asthma	First episode of otitis media at < 6 months
Stark et al. (2003)	499 children of parents with asthma or allergies	Any lower respiratory tract infection[b]

Dampness or mould measure	Risk estimate (95% CI)
Building dampness	3.14 (1.01–9.80)

Dampness or mould measure	Risk estimate (95% CI)
Exposure to visible mould:	
None	1.0
Low	1.5 (1.1-2.3)
High	5.1 (2.2-12.1)
Mould	1.37 (0.91–2.02)
Penicillium:	
undetectable	1.00
1–499 CFU/m³	0.75 (0.52–1.08)
500–999 CFU/m³	1.89 (0.67–5.30)
≥ 1000 CFU/m³	1.27 (0.56–2.86)
Cladosporium:	
undetectable	1.00
1–499 CFU/m³	1.04 (0.70–1.56)
500–999 CFU/m³	0.92 (0.48–1.79)
≥ 1000 CFU/m³	1.09 (0.52–2.29)
Other mould:	
undetectable	1.00
1–499 CFU/m³	1.21 (0.84–1.74)
500–999 CFU/m³	0.72 (0.29–1.80)
≥ 1000 CFU/m³	3.45 (1.36–8.76)

Dampness or mould measure	Risk estimate (95% CI)
Water damage: mould or mildew	1.34 (0.99–1.82)
Fungal exposure: high (in 90th percentile of distribution) *vs* low	
Airborne:	
Aspergillus	0.99 (0.58–1.68)
Cladosporium	1.17 (0.77–1.77)
Penicillium	1.73 (1.23–2.43)
Yeasts	0.80 (0.47–1.38)
Dust-borne:	
Alternaria	1.51 (1.00–2.28)
Aspergillus	0.94 (0.54–1.65)
Aureobasidium	1.21 (0.76–1.93)
Cladosporium	1.52 (1.02–2.25)
Coelomyces	1.09 (0.66–1.79)

▶

Reference	Participants	Outcome
		Lower respiratory tract infection without wheeze
		Lower respiratory tract infection with wheeze
Müller et al. (2002)	475 premature infants and newborns at risk of atopy	Respiratory tract infections
Cross-sectional studies		
du Prel et al. (2006)	22 666 children (aged 6 years) in eastern Germany	> 4 colds in past 12 months
	6222 children (aged 6 years) in western Germany	> 4 colds in past 12 months

Dampness or mould measure	Risk estimate (95% CI)
Fusarium	1.28 (0.79–2.09)
Penicillium	1.07 (0.61–1.86)
Ulocladium	1.24 (0.83–1.85)
Wallemia	0.92 (0.54–1.57)
Yeasts	0.93 (0.55–1.57)
Zygomyetes	1.96 (1.35–2.83)
Airborne:	
Aspergillus	0.80 (0.26–2.44)
Cladosporium	1.33 (0.61–2.91)
Penicillium	3.32 (1.83–6.04)
Yeasts	0.73 (0.28–1.91)
Dust-borne:	
Alternaria	1.12 (0.44–2.88)
Aspergillus	1.80 (0.86–3.76)
Aureobasidium	0.85 (0.28–2.56)
Cladosporium	1.68 (0.78–3.60)
Fusarium	1.13 (0.44–2.90)
Penicillium	0.62 (0.16–2.43)
Yeasts	1.77 (0.85–3.71)
Zygomyetes	1.19 (0.47–3.00)
Water damage: mould or mildew	1.35 (0.90–2.04)
Airborne:	
Aspergillus	1.05 (0.55–2.01)
Cladosporium	1.13 (0.64–2.00)
Penicillium	1.56 (0.92–2.65)
Yeasts	0.78 (0.38–1.60)
Dust-borne:	
Alternaria	1.82 (1.08–3.08)
Aspergillus	0.47 (0.16–1.41)
Aureobasidium	1.42 (0.80–2.50)
Cladosporium	1.57 (0.91–2.69)
Coelomyces	0.82 (0.36–1.88)
Fusarium	1.35 (0.71–2.57)
Penicillium	1.28 (0.67–2.47)
Ulocladium	1.33 (0.76–2.35)
Wallemia	0.46 (0.15–1.36)
Yeasts	0.53 (0.21–1.35)
Zygomyetes	2.60 (1.63–4.16)
Indoor exposure to *Penicillium* spores > 100 CFU/m^3	6.88 (1.21–38.9)
Damp housing conditions	1.41 (1.25–1.60)
Damp housing conditions	1.62 (1.21–2.17)

Reference	Participants	Outcome
Karevold et al. (2006)	3406 children (aged 10 years)	Otitis media Lower respiratory tract infections
Spengler et al. (2004)	5951 children (aged 8–12 years)	Current upper respiratory tract infection
Yang et al. (1997a)	4164 primary-school children (aged 6–12 years)	Pneumonia
Nafstad et al. (2005)	942 children (aged 3–5 years) attending day-care centres	Common cold Pharyngitis or tonsillitis Otitis media Bronchitis Pneumonia

Current asthma

Adults
Prospective studies

Matheson et al. (2005)	845 adults (aged 20–45 years)	Asthma attack in past 12 months

Cross-sectional studies

Dharmage et al. (2001)	485 participants in follow-up study to ECRHS	Bronchial hyperreactivity only
Gunnbjörnsdottir et al. (2006)	15 995 adults (aged 20–44 years) who participated in the ECRHS	Asthma onset
Skorge et al. (2005)	2401 adults (aged 26–82 years)	Asthma
Zock et al. (2002)	18 873 people in 38 study centres of the ECRHS	Current asthma Bronchial responsiveness Current asthma Bronchial responsiveness Current asthma Bronchial responsiveness

Dampness or mould measure	Risk estimate (95% CI)
Dampness at home	1.2 (1.0–1.5) 1.3 (1.0–1.7)
Water damage Presence of moulds	1.23 (0.98–1.55) 1.74 (1.35–2.25)
Dampness at home	1.85 (0.94–3.61)
Dampness problems	1.08 (0.64–1.81) 0.98 (0.67–1.42) 1.00 (0.70–1.43) 1.52 (0.78–2.96) 0.65 (0.26–1.62)
Ergosterol[a] Total fungi[a] Other fungi[a] *Cladosporium*[a]	0.92 (0.59–1.44) 1.54 (0.98–2.43) 1.23 (0.92–1.66) 1.52 (1.08–2.13)
Levels of *Cladosporium* in highest quartile Levels of *Penicillium* in highest quartile	8.5 (1.6–44.3) 3.9 (1.1–14.3)
Water damage Wet floors Visible moulds Any dampness	1.18 (0.95–1.44) 1.67 (1.22–2.27) 1.53 (1.18–1.98) 1.27 (1.06–1.52)
Mould: only earlier Mould: earlier and last year Water damage: only earlier Water damage: earlier and last year	1.4 (0.68–2.85) 1.4 (0.78–2.62) 1.4 (0.78–2.62) 1.2 (0.49–2.85
Water damage in past year	1.13 (0.95–1.35) 1.15 (0.97–1.35)
Water on basement floor	1.54 (0.84–2.82) 1.05 (0.71–1.55)
Mould or mildew in past year	1.28 (1.13–1.46) 1.14 (1.01–1.29)

Reference	Participants	Outcome
Children *Cross-sectional studies*		
Bornehag et al. (2005)	10 851 preschool children (aged 1–6 years)	Doctor-diagnosed asthma
Simoni et al. (2005)	20 016 children (mean age 7 years) and 13 266 adolescents (mean age 13 years)	Children: asthma only current Children: asthma only early Children: asthma both Adolescents: asthma only current Adolescents: asthma only early Adolescents: asthma both
Tavernier et al. (2006)	105 children with asthma and 95 children without asthma	Asthma
Rönmark et al. (1999)	Schoolchildren (aged 7–8 years) (3431 questionnaire; 2149 skin test)	Non-atopic asthma Atopic asthma
Yang et al. (1997b)[c]	4164 primary-school children (aged 6–12 years)	Asthma
Yang et al. (1997a)[c]	4164 primary-school children (aged 6–12 years)	Asthma
Forsberg et al. (1997)	15 962 children (aged 6–12 years)	Asthma treatment
Spengler et al. (2004)	5951 children (8–12 years)	Current doctor-diagnosed asthma
Wickens et al. (1999)	474 children (aged 7–9 years) in the International Study of Asthma and Allergies in Childhood	Asthma
Dales, Miller, White (1999)	403 elementary-school children	Asthma
Li, Hsu (1996)	1340 children (aged 8–12 years)	Asthma

Dampness or mould measure	Risk estimate (95% CI)
Water leakage	1.28 (1.04–1.58)
Floor moisture	1.39 (1.00–1.93)
Visible dampness	2.14 (1.09–4.24)
Condensation on window	1.50 (1.16–1.94)
Mould or dampness	1.39 (1.00–1.93)
	1.80 (1.41–2.30)
	1.17 (0.80–1.71)
	1.28 (0.90–1.82)
	1.89 (1.38–2.59)
	1.62 (1.00–2.62)
Self-reported dampness in kitchen and bathroom	2.72 (0.50–14.8)
Self-reported absence of dampness at home [d]	0.36 (0.14–0.91)
Dampness at home	1.78 (1.10–2.89)
	1.40 (0.81–2.42)
Dampness at home	1.68 (1.16–2.43)
Dampness at home	1.73 (1.20–2.49)
Moisture stains or mould: current exposure	0.9 (0.7–1.2)
Moisture stains or mould: during child's first 2 years	2.0 (1.6–2.6)
Water damage	1.37 (0.69–2.70)
Presence of mould	2.82 (1.63–4.88)
Mould	12.99 (2.63–64.2)
Aspergillus (indoor source fungi)	0.92 (0.35–2.44)
Alternaria (indoor source fungi)	1.90 (0.55–6.59)
Cladosporium (outdoor source fungi)	0.46 (0.18–1.21)
Epicoccum (outdoor source fungi)	0.88 (0.30–2.57)
Yeast (outdoor source fungi)	2.16 (0.73–6.39)
Ergosterol	1.3 (0.6–2.8)
Self-reported dampness	1.25 (0.81–1.95)
Dampness	1.18 (0.70–1.98)
Mould	1.18 (0.70–1.98)
Stuffy odour	1.05 (0.66–1.66)
Water damage	1.95 (0.80–4.76)
Flooding	0.94 (0.50–1.74)

TABLE A1.2. CONT.

Reference	Participants	Outcome
Nafstad et al. (2005)	942 children (aged 3–5 years) attending day-care centres	Asthma
Peters et al. (1999)	3676 children	Current asthma

Adults and children
Cross-sectional studies

Salo et al. (2006)	2456 adults and children	Current doctor-diagnosed asthma

Upper respiratory tract symptoms (excluding allergic rhinitis)

Adults
Cross-sectional studies

Haverinen et al. (2001)	1017 adults	Prolonged rhinitis Impaired sense of smell Nasal bleeding Sore throat Hoarseness
		Prolonged rhinitis Impaired sense of smell Nasal bleeding Sore throat Hoarseness
		Prolonged rhinitis Impaired sense of smell

Dampness or mould measure	Risk estimate (95% CI)
Dampness problems	0.76 (0.40–1.42)
Water damage	1.27 ($p \geq 0.15$)
Mildew	1.17 ($p \geq 0.15$)
Alternaria alternata concentration, adjusted model:	
1st tertile	1.00
2nd tertile	1.52 (0.90–2.55
3rd tertile	1.84 (1.18–2.85)
Alternaria alternata concentration, adjusted model including other indoor allergens:	
1st tertile	1.00
2nd tertile	1.56 (0.96–2.53)
3rd tertile	1.89 (1.25–2.85)
Alternaria alternata concentration, adjusted model including other indoor allergens and dust weight:	
1st tertile	1.00
2nd tertile	1.55 (0.96–2.52)
3rd tertile	1.86 (1.22–2.84)
Alternaria alternata concentration, adjusted model including other indoor allergens, dust weight and endotoxins:	
1st tertile	1.00
2nd tertile	1.45 (0.88–2.39)
3rd tertile	1.73 (1.08–2.77)
Visible mould growth or mould odour at home *vs* neither	1.00 (0.73–1.35)
	1.35 (0.66–2.76)
	0.51 (0.18–1.47)
	1.27 (0.64–2.51)
	1.59 (0.82–3.07)
Grade I[e]	1.00
	1.00
	1.00
	1.00
	1.00
Grade II[e]	1.05 (0.71–1.55)
	1.09 (0.44–2.67)

▶

TABLE A1.2. CONT.

Reference	Participants	Outcome
		Nasal bleeding Sore throat Hoarseness
		Prolonged rhinitis Impaired sense of smell Nasal bleeding Sore throat Hoarseness
Haverinen-Shaughnessy et al. (2007)	81 randomly selected elementary-school teachers	Blocked nose, today Blocked nose, this week Sore throat, this week
		Blocked nose, today Blocked nose, this week Sore throat, this week
		Blocked nose, today Blocked nose, this week Sore throat, this week
		Blocked nose, today Blocked nose, this week Sore throat, this week
		Blocked nose, today Blocked nose, this week Sore throat, this week
		Blocked nose, today Blocked nose, this week Sore throat, this week
		Blocked nose, today Blocked nose, this week Sore throat, this week
		Blocked nose, today Blocked nose, this week Sore throat, this week
		Blocked nose, today Blocked nose, this week Sore throat, this week
Park et al. (2004)	323 employees in 13 college buildings	Nasal symptoms Sinus symptoms Throat irritation

Dampness or mould measure	Risk estimate (95% CI)
	0.73 (0.18–2.88)
	1.64 (0.74–3.63)
	1.38 (0.61–3.13)
Grade III[e]	1.03 (0.68–1.57)
	0.88 (0.34–2.33)
	0.83 (0.20–3.36)
	1.09 (0.45–2.65)
	2.06 (0.88–4.84)
Total fungi, adjusted[f]	1.26 (0.87–1.83)
	1.05 (0.71–1.54)
	0.54 (0.33–0.89)
Viable fungi, MEA, adjusted[f]	0.91 (0.70–1.18)
	1.07 (0.84–1.35)
	0.75 (0.56–1.01)
Viable fungi, DG18, adjusted[f]	0.96 (0.76–1.22)
	1.07 (0.87–1.32)
	0.69 (0.49–0.97)
Total fungi, adjusted[g]	1.05 (0.75–1.45)
	0.98 (0.70–1.38)
	0.87 (0.60–1.25)
Viable fungi, MEA, adjusted[g]	0.79 (0.63–0.99)
	0.72 (0.57–0.90)
	0.70 (0.52–0.95)
Viable fungi, DG-18, adjusted[g]	0.81 (0.65–1.01)
	0.79 (0.63–0.98)
	0.81 (0.63–1.03)
Total fungi, adjusted[h]	1.02 (0.64–1.62)
	0.93 (0.56–1.54)
	1.03 (0.62–1.71)
Viable fungi, MEA, adjusted[h]	0.95 (0.61–1.47)
	0.86 (0.58–1.27)
	1.13 (0.76–1.68)
Viable fungi, DG-18, adjusted[h]	0.81 (0.50–1.31)
	0.72 (0.49–1.08)
	0.95 (0.63–1.44)
Water stains: continuous variable	1.5 (0.8–2.8)
	1.6 (0.9–2.9)
	2.4 (1.3–4.4)

▶

Reference	Participants	Outcome
		Nasal symptoms
		Sinus symptoms
		Throat irritation
		Nasal symptoms
		Sinus symptoms
		Throat irritation
		Nasal symptoms
		Sinus symptoms
		Throat irritation
		Nasal symptoms
		Sinus symptoms
		Throat irritation
		Nasal symptoms
		Sinus symptoms
		Throat irritation
		Nasal symptoms
		Sinus symptoms
		Throat irritation
Park et al. (2006)	888 occupants of a water-damaged building	Throat irritation
Bakke et al. (2007)	173 staff in four university buildings	Nasal symptoms
		Dry throat
Dales, Burnett, Zwanenburg (1991)	14 799 parents of school-aged children (aged 5–8 years)	Upper respiratory tract symptoms
Ruotsalainen, Jaakkola, Jaakkola (1995)	268 female day-care workers	Mucosal symptoms
		Allergic symptoms
		Mucosal symptoms
		Allergic symptoms

Children
Cross-sectional studies

Reference	Participants	Outcome
Bornehag et al. (2005)	10 851 preschool children (aged 1–6 years)	Rhinitis in past 12 months
		Rhinitis (doctor-diagnosed)
		Rhinitis in past 12 months
		Rhinitis (doctor-diagnosed)
		Rhinitis in past 12 months
		Rhinitis (doctor-diagnosed)
		Rhinitis in past 12 months
		Rhinitis (doctor-diagnosed)

Dampness or mould measure	Risk estimate (95% CI)
Water stains: any	4.4 (1.2–15.3)
	3.8 (1.1–13.4)
	2.0 (0.7–5.6)
Any visible mould	1.7 (1.0–3.0)
	2.0 (1.2–3.4)
	1.3 (0.7–2.1)
Any mould odour	1.1 (0.6–2.1)
	1.3 (0.7–2.5)
	2.3 (1.2–4.3)
Any damp material or standing water	1.7 (0.5–6.0)
	0.8 (0.2–2.9)
	1.5 (0.4–5.1)
Factor combinations, weighted for water stains	2.4 (1.3–4.6)
	1.8 (1.0–3.4)
	1.6 (0.9–3.0)
Factor combinations, weighted for visible mould	2.5 (1.3–4.7)
	2.2 (1.2–4.1)
	1.5 (0.8–2.8)
Fungi[i]	1.4 (0.93–2.09)
Fungi high, endotoxin low[j]	1.5 (0.77–3.01)
Fungi low, endotoxin high[j]	1.6 (0.79–3.34)
Fungi high, endotoxin high[j]	2.2 (1.20–3.90)
Building dampness	0.42 (0.11–1.65)
	0.80 (0.17–3.72)
Dampness or mould	1.50 (1.30–1.61)
Low exposure to water damage, no mould odour	0.55 (0.26–1.17)
	0.41 (0.19–0.89)
High exposure to water damage, mould odour	1.63 (0.69–3.84)
	1.66 (0.71–3.89)
Water leakage	1.35 (1.12–1.62)
	1.23 (0.83–1.82)
Floor moisture	1.75 (1.39–2.21)
	1.46 (0.88–2.41)
Visible dampness	1.67 (0.94–2.96)
	2.95 (1.15–7.59)
Condensation on window	1.60 (1.32–1.94)
	1.49 (1.00–2.23)

Reference	Participants	Outcome
Kuyucu et al. (2006)	2774 children (aged 9–11 years)	Current rhinitis
du Prel et al. (2006)	22 666 children (aged 6 years) in eastern Germany	Sneeze attacks in past 12 months
	6222 children (aged 6 years) in western Germany	Sneeze attacks in past 12 months
Prospective studies		
Simoni et al. (2005)	20 016 children (mean age 7 years)	Rhinoconjunctivitis: never Rhinoconjunctivitis: only current Rhinoconjunctivitis: only early Rhinoconjunctivitis: both
Retrospective studies		
Andriessen, Brunekreef, Roemer (1998)	1614 children with symptoms of asthma and chronic cough	Prevalence of upper respiratory tract symptoms

Allergic rhinitis

Children
Prospective studies

Reference	Participants	Outcome
Biagini et al. (2006)	633 infants enrolled in Cincinnati Childhood Allergen and Air Pollution Study with at least one parent with positive skin-prick test	Allergic rhinitis
Stark PC et al. (2005)	405 children of parents with asthma or allergies	Allergic rhinitis

Dampness or mould measure	Risk estimate (95% CI)
Dampness or mould at 1 year of age	1.70 (1.25–2.31)
Damp housing conditions	1.52 (1.26–1.83)
Damp housing conditions	2.25 (1.52–3.33)

Mould or dampness	1.00
	1.03 (0.72–1.49)
	1.46 (1.13–1.89)
	1.46 (1.01–2.09)

Moisture stains	1.03 (0.91–1.17)
Mould	1.00 (0.86–1.16)

Exposure to visible mould:	
None	1.0
Low	1.2 (0.6–2.5)
High	3.2 (0.7–14.8)

Fungal exposure: high (in 90th percentile of distribution) *vs* low

Airborne:	
Aspergillus	1.10 (0.43–2.80)
Cladosporium	1.25 (0.43–3.64)
Non-sporulating	0.55 (0.17–1.81)
Penicillium	0.69 (0.23–2.06)
Yeasts	0.79 (0.24–2.60)
Total	0.83 (0.28–2.43)

Dust-borne:	
Alternaria	2.34 (1.12–4.91)
Aspergillus	2.57 (1.22–5.40)
Aureobasidium	3.12 (1.50–6.50)
Cladosporium	1.88 (0.81–4.35)
Dust-borne, *Coelomyces*	0.93 (0.36–2.38)
Fusarium	1.81 (0.76–4.34)
Non-sporulating	2.45 (1.15–5.22)
Penicillium	1.51 (0.63–3.64)
Ulocladium	1.04 (0.37–2.95)
Wallemia	1.73 (0.80–3.75)
Yeasts	2.90 (1.37–6.09)
Zygomyetes	0.87 (0.31–2.44)
Total	3.13 (1.51–6.47)

▶

TABLE A1.2. CONT.

Reference	Participants	Outcome

Cross-sectional studies

Reference	Participants	Outcome
Li, Hsu (1996)	1340 children (aged 8–12 years)	Allergic rhinitis
Yang et al. (1997b)	4164 primary-school children (aged 6–12 years)	Allergic rhinitis
Li, Hsu (1997)	46 children (aged 7–15 years)	Allergic rhinitis
Zacharasiewicz et al. (1999)	18 606 children (aged 6–9 years)	Atopic rhinitis

Dampness or mould measure	Risk estimate (95% CI)
Water damage, mould or mildew in year 1:	
Model 1[k]	1.66 (0.88–3.15)
Model 2[l]	1.77 (0.94–3.34)
Model 3[m]	1.66 (0.87–3.17)
Dust-borne *Alternaria*:	
Model 1[k]	1.40 (0.61–3.23)
Model 2[l]	1.52 (0.67–3.44)
Model 3[m]	2.07 (0.98–4.37)
Dust-borne *Aspergillus*:	
Model 1[k]	3.27 (1.50–7.14)
Model 2[l]	2.93 (1.36–6.30)
Model 3[m]	2.73 (1.27–5.87)
Dust-borne *Aureobasidium*:	
Model 1[k]	3.04 (1.33–6.93)
Model 2[l]	3.06 (1.35–6.91)
Dust-borne yeasts:	
Model 1[k]	2.67 (1.26–5.66)
Model 2[l]	2.80 (1.33–5.93)
Model 3[m]	2.52 (1.18-5.36)

Self-reported dampness	1.39 (1.05–1.84)
Dampness	1.56 (1.11–2.18)
Mould	1.56 (1.11–2.18)
Stuffy odour	1.37 (1.03–1.83)
Water damage	1.47 (0.73–2.97)
Flooding	1.55 (1.08–2.23)

Dampness at home	1.52 (1.25–1.85)

Self-reported dampness	3.50 (1.00–12.34)
Mould	3.50 (1.00–12.34)
Water damage	0.73 (0.23–2.37)
Stuffy odour	2.73 (0.77–9.69)
Flooding	1.92 (0.38–9.76)
Dampness	2.09 (0.47–9.38)

Dampness at home	1.51 (1.31–1.74)

Reference	Participants	Outcome
Cough		
Adults		
Cross-sectional studies		
Haverinen-Shaughnessy et al. (2007)	81 randomly selected elementary-school teachers	Cough, today Cough, this week
		Cough, today Cough, this week
		Cough, today Cough, this week
		Cough, today Cough, this week
		Cough, today Cough, this week
		Cough, today Cough, this week
		Cough, today Cough, this week
		Cough, today Cough, this week
		Cough, today Cough, this week
Brunekreef (1992)	3344 parents of children (aged 6–12 years)	Women, cough Men, cough
Gunnbjörnsdottir et al. (2006)	15 995 adults (aged 20– 44 years) who participated in the ECRHS	Nocturnal cough Productive cough
		Nocturnal cough Productive cough
		Nocturnal cough Productive cough
		Nocturnal cough Productive cough
		Nocturnal cough Productive cough

Dampness or mould measure	Risk estimate (95% CI)
Total fungi: adjusted[f]	1.11 (0.72–1.70) 1.10 (0.78–1.55)
Viable fungi: MEA, adjusted[f]	0.77 (0.55–1.09) 0.83 (0.65–1.05)
Viable fungi: DG18, adjusted[f]	0.65 (0.48–0.89) 0.81 (0.65–1.02)
Total fungi: adjusted[g]	0.96 (0.69–1.34) 0.87 (0.66–1.13)
Viable fungi: MEA, adjusted[g]	0.57 (0.37–0.89) 0.77 (0.60–1.00)
Viable fungi: DG18, adjusted[g]	0.74 (0.54–1.03) 0.82 (0.66–1.01)
Total fungi: adjusted[h]	1.09 (0.62–1.91) 0.87 (0.53–1.44)
Viable fungi: MEA, adjusted[h]	0.91 (0.53–1.55) 0.78 (0.50–1.21)
Viable fungi: DG18, adjusted[h]	0.71 (0.38–1.32) 0.59 (0.36–0.99)
Damp stains or mould	1.75 (1.30–2.36) 2.56 (1.94–3.38)
Water damage	1.34 (1.21–1.49) 1.34 (1.18–1.51)
Wet floors	1.66 (1.38–2.00) 1.52 (1.23–1.87)
Visible mould	1.41 (1.22–1.63) 1.36 (1.15–1.61)
Any dampness	1.40 (1.28–1.54) 1.34 (1.20–1.50)
Onset in damp homes Remission in damp homes	1.26 (1.13–1.41) 0.84 (0.73–0.97)

TABLE A1.2. CONT.

Reference	Participants	Outcome
Skorge et al. (2005)	2401 adults (aged 26–82 years)	Cough with phlegm Chronic cough
		Cough with phlegm Chronic cough
		Cough with phlegm Chronic cough
		Cough with phlegm Chronic cough
		Cough with phlegm Chronic cough
Haverinen et al. (2001)	1017 adults	Cough without phlegm Cough with phlegm Cough
		Cough without phlegm Cough with phlegm Cough
		Cough without phlegm Cough with phlegm Cough
		Cough without phlegm Cough with phlegm Cough
Park et al. (2004)	323 employees in 13 college buildings	Cough
Gunnbjörnsdottir et al. (2003)	1853 young adults (aged 20–44 years)	Nocturnal cough Long-term cough
		Nocturnal cough Long-term cough
		Nocturnal cough Long-term cough

Dampness or mould measure	Risk estimate (95% CI)
Mould: only earlier	1.6 (1.01–2.38)
	1.2 (0.71–2.19)
Mould: earlier and last year	1.7 (1.08–2.64)
	1.2 (1.17–2.48)
Water damage: only earlier	1.2 (0.84–1.72)
	1.2 (0.74–1.86)
Water damage: earlier and last year	1.2 (0.74–2.01)
	1.2 (0.61–2.19)
Mould	AF=3.4 (1.0–5.9)
	AF=3.9 (0.0–7.6)
Visible mould growth or odour at home *vs* neither	1.52 (1.04–2.22)
	1.02 (0.72–1.43)
	1.12 (0.64–1.97)
Grade I[e]	1.00
	1.00
	1.00
Grade II[e]	1.23 (0.76–1.98)
	0.79 (0.50–1.24)
	0.81 (0.38–1.73)
Grade III[e]	1.52 (0.94–2.47)
	1.10 (0.70–1.73)
	1.04 (0.48–2.21)
Water stains: continuous variable	1.3 (0.6–2.6)
Water stains: any	3.2 (0.7–14.4)
Any visible mould	1.5 (0.8–2.8)
Any mould odour	1.7 (0.8–3.6)
Any damp material or standing water	1.0 (0.2–4.5)
Factor combinations, weighted for water stains	1.5 (0.7–3.2)
Factor combinations, weighted for visible mould	1.7 (0.8–3.6)
Only mould	1.21 (0.90–1.64)
	1.10 (0.74–1.61)
Only water damage	1.67 (0.93–2.98)
	1.46 (0.72–2.94)
Mould and water damage	1.18 (0.68–2.04)
	2.23 (1.24–4.00)

Reference	Participants	Outcome
Ruotsalainen, Jaakkola, Jaakkola (1995)	268 female day-care workers	Cough
Children *Cross-sectional studies*		
Bornehag et al. (2005)	10 851 preschool children (aged 1–6 years)	Nocturnal cough in past 12 months

Simoni et al. (2005)	20 016 children (mean age 7 years) and 13 266 adolescents (mean age 13 years)	Children, persistent cough or phlegm:
		    Never
		    Only current
		    Only early
		    Both
		Adolescents, persistent cough or phlegm:
		    Never
		    Only current
		    Only early
		    Both

Forsberg et al. (1997)	15 962 children (aged 6–12 years)	Dry cough
Li, Hsu (1996)	1340 children (aged 8–12 years)	Cough
Mommers et al. (2005)	1191 children (aged 7–8 yeas)	Cough
Peters et al. (1999)	3676 children	Cough
Spengler et al. (2004)	5951 children (aged 8–12 years)	Persistent cough Current dry cough Persistent dry cough Persistent cough Current dry cough Persistent dry cough

Dampness or mould measure	Risk estimate (95% CI)
Water damage, no mould odour	1.10 (0.17–6.96)
Water damage and mould odour	2.23 (0.31–15.8)
Water leakage	1.22 (1.01–1.47)
Floor moisture	1.45 (1.09–1.93)
Visible dampness	2.50 (1.63–3.82)
Condensation on window	1.61 (1.28–2.02)
Mould or dampness	
	1.00
	1.86 (1.19–2.91)
	1.89 (1.31–2.71)
	1.64 (0.96–2.79)
	1.00
	1.19 (0.74–1.91)
	0.80 (0.46–1.40)
	1.48 (0.78–2.81)
Moisture stains or mould: current	1.6 (1.3–1.9)
Moisture stains or mould: during child's first 2 years	1.6 (1.3–2.0)
Self-reported dampness	2.52 (1.34–4.75)
Dampness	1.43 (0.067–3.05)
Mould	1.87 (1.00–3.25)
Stuffy odour	1.66 (0.89–3.11)
Water damage	5.74 (2.20–14.95)
Flooding	1.41 (0.64–3.14)
Mould or damp spots: short period	2.03 (1.32–3.14)
Mould or damp spots: long period	3.25 (1.35–8.28)
Mould or damp spots: always	1.24 (0.40–3.88)
Water damage	1.38 ($p < 0.15$)
Mildew	1.45 ($p < 0.05$)
Water damage	1.51 (1.06–2.16)
	1.35 (1.08–1.69)
	1.33 (0.85–2.09)
Presence of mould	1.88 (1.35–2.63)
	1.40 (1.12–1.76)
	1.53 (0.99–2.35)

TABLE A1.2. CONT.

Reference	Participants	Outcome
Strachan, Elton (1986)	165 children (aged 7–8 years)	Nocturnal cough
Yang et al. (1997b)[c]	4164 primary-school children (aged 6–12 years)	Cough
Yang et al. (1997a)[c]	4164 primary-school children (aged 6–12 years)	Cough
Yangzong et al. (2006)	2026 children (aged 12–14 years) living at > 3900 m	Nocturnal cough
du Prel et al. (2006)	22 666 children (aged 6 years) in eastern Germany 6222 children (aged 6 years) in western Germany	Frequent cough Frequent cough
Cuijpers et al. (1995)	470 primary-school children (aged 6–12 years)	Chronic cough, boys Chronic cough, girls

Wheeze

Adults
Cross-sectional studies

Strachan, Carey (1995)	961 secondary-school students; 486 cases 475 controls	Frequent attacks of wheeze Speech-limiting wheeze Frequent speech-limiting wheeze
Nriagu et al. (1999)	693 adults	Wheeze
Dharmage et al. (2001)	485 participants in follow-up study to the ECRHS	Wheeze only

Dampness or mould measure	Risk estimate (95% CI)
Damp	4.0[n] ($p < 0.001$)
Mould	4.8[n] ($p < 0.001$)
Dampness at home	1.65 (1.36–2.00)
Dampness at home	1.71 (1.42–2.06)
Dampness problems	2.1 (1.3–3.5)
Damp housing conditions	1.66 (1.42–1.95)
Damp housing conditions	2.60 (1.90–3.55)
Mould growth	
Sometimes	2.26 (0.83–6.15)
Often	1.59 (0.28–9.11)
Always	3.36 (0.80–14.10)
Mould growth	
Sometimes	0.21 (0.03–1.79)
Often	(Not estimated)
Always	0.79 (0.07–8.34)

No bedroom damp or mould	1.00
Damp only	1.19
Damp with mould	1.69
No bedroom damp or mould	1.00
Damp only	1.04
Damp with mould	2.36 ($p < 0.05$)
No bedroom damp or mould	1.00
Damp only	Not defined
Damp with mould	2.55 ($p < 0.05$)
Dampness at home	2.13 (0.95–4.75)
Ergosterol levels in upper three quartiles *vs* first quartile	Range: 3.6–4.7 (all $p < 0.05$)

TABLE A1.2. CONT.

Reference	Participants	Outcome
Park et al. (2004)	323 employees in 13 college buildings	Wheeze
Brunekreef (1992)	3344 parents of children aged 6–12 years	Wheeze
Gunnbjörnsdottir et al. (2006)	15 995 adults (aged 20–44 years) who participated in the ECRHS	Wheeze
Rennie et al. (2005)	1998 adults (aged 18–74 years)	Wheeze with shortness of breath
Skorge et al. (2005)	2401 adults (aged 26–82 years)	Wheeze
Haverinen et al. (2001)	1017 adults	Wheeze
Ruotsalainen, Jaakkola, Jaakkola (1995)	268 female day-care workers	Chronic wheeze
Zock et al. (2002)	18 873 people in 38 study centres of the ECRHS	Wheeze and breathlessness in past year Wheeze apart from colds in past year Wheeze and breathlessness in past year Wheeze apart from colds in past year Wheeze and breathlessness in past year Wheeze apart from colds in past year

Dampness or mould measure	Risk estimate (95% CI)
Water stains: continuous variable	2.3 (1.1–4.5)
Water stains: any	2.6 (0.7–9.2)
Any visible mould	2.0 (1.1–3.7)
Any mould odour	1.1 (0.5–2.3)
Any damp material or standing water	1.2 (0.3–4.5)
Factor combinations: weighted for water stains	1.8 (0.9–3.5)
Factor combinations: weighted for visible mould	1.7 (0.9–3.4)
Damp stains or mould	1.43 (1.15–1.77), women
	1.63 (1.30–2.06), men
Water damage	1.32 (1.17–1.49)
Wet floor	1.54 (1.25–1.90)
Visible mould	1.54 (1.31–1.80)
Any dampness	1.38 (1.24–1.53)
Onset in damp homes	1.28 (1.12–1.46)
Remission in damp homes	0.88 (0.74–1.03)
Damp housing	1.29 (0.62–2.67), men
	1.85 (1.08–3.17), women
Mould: only earlier	1.5 (0.99–2.34)
Mould: earlier and last year	1.3 (0.92–1.86)
Water damage: only earlier	1.3 (0.92–1.86)
Water damage: earlier and last year	1.0 (0.61–1.69)
Mould	AF = 4.7 (2.0–7.2)
Visible mould growth or odour at home vs neither	0.83 (0.43–1.60)
Grade I[e]	1.00
Grade II[e]	0.44 (0.14–1.34)
Grade III[e]	1.52 (0.67–3.47)
Water damage, no mould odour	1.66 (0.72–3.82)
Water damage and mould odour	1.28 (0.44–3.73)
Water damage in past year	
	1.16 (1.00–1.34)
	1.23 (1.06–1.44)
Water on basement floor	
	1.46 (1.07–2.01)
	1.26 (0.81–1.98)
Mould or mildew in past year	
	1.34 (1.18–1.51)
	1.44 (1.30–1.60)

Reference	Participants	Outcome
Children *Prospective studies*		
Dales et al. (2006)	332 children	Number of days with wheeze per year
Emenius et al. (2004a)	540 infants (aged 2 years) 181 cases with recurrent wheeze 359 controls	Recurrent wheeze (3 or more episodes after 3 months of age) plus either use of inhaled steroids or symptoms suggestive of bronchial hyperreactivity
Emenius et al. (2004b)	540 infants (aged 2 years) 181 cases with recurrent wheeze 359 controls	Recurrent wheeze (3 or more episodes after 3 months of age) plus either use of inhaled steroids or symptoms suggestive of bronchial hyperreactivity
Douwes et al. (2006)	696 children with atopic mothers	Wheeze: in past 12 months Wheeze: early transient in past 4 years Wheeze: persistent in past 4 years Wheeze: in past 12 months Wheeze: early transient in past 4 years Wheeze: persistent in past 4 years Wheeze: in past 12 months Wheeze: early transient in past 4 years Wheeze: persistent in past 4 years Wheeze: in past 12 months Wheeze: early transient in past 4 years Wheeze: persistent in past 4 years

Dampness or mould measure	Risk estimate (95% CI)
Endotoxins:	
1st tertile	2.28 (4.55)°
2nd tertile	4.26 (10.1)
3rd tertile	5.66 (12.4)
Absolute indoor humidity > median, 5.8 g/kg	1.7 (1.0–2.9)
Relative humidity > 45%	0.8 (0.4–1.5)
Window pane condensation (on four questionnaires)	2.2 (1.1–4.5)
Any dampness	1.4 (0.9–2.2)
Mould odour	2.0 (1.0–3.9
Mould spots on surface material or tile joints in wet areas	
(shower or bathroom)	1.0 (0.5–1.7)
Any other sign of dampness	1.6 (1.0–2.5)
Any other sign of dampness combined with reported window pane	
condensation > 2 times, absolute indoor humidity level > 5.8 g/m³	2.0 (1.2–3.4)
Prospectively reported dampness or noted at inspection	1.5 (1.0–2.3)
Sign of dampness both prospectively and at time of inspection	1.8 (0.9–3.5)
Window pane condensation	
(on all 3 questionnaires and inspection form)	2.2 (1.1–4.5)
Damage by damp	1.4 (1.1–1.8)
Mould odour	1.6 (1.1–2.3)
Visible mould last year	1.5 (1.0–2.2)
Any sign of dampness	1.4 (1.1–1.8)
1 of 3 signs of dampness	1.2 (0.9–1.7)
2 of 3 signs of dampness	1.5 (1.0–2.4)
3 of 3 signs of dampness	2.2 (1.3–4.2)
Glucan: medium	1.50 (0.77–2.94)
	0.89 (0.46–1.71)
	1.16 (0.52–2.62)
Glucan: high	0.76 (0.34–1.72)
	0.57 (0.28–1.16)
	0.43 (0.15–1.21)
Extracellular *Aspergillus* or *Penicillium* polysaccharides: medium	1.28 (0.70–2.32)
	0.99 (0.56–1.76)
	1.07 (0.53–2.16)
Extracellular *Aspergillus* or *Penicillium* polysaccharides: high	0.63 (0.30–1.32)
	0.67 (0.36–1.23)
	0.37 (0.15–0.96)

TABLE A1.2. CONT.

Reference	Participants	Outcome
Cho et al. (2006)	640 infants of at least one atopic parent	Recurrent wheeze
		Recurrent wheeze combined with any allergen
Cross-sectional studies		
Bornehag et al. (2005)	10 851 preschool children (aged 1–6 years)	Wheeze
Simoni et al. (2005)	20 016 children (mean age 7 years) 13 266 adolescents (mean age 13 years)	Children, wheeze: Never Only current Only earlier Both Adolescents, wheeze: Never Only current Only earlier Both
Li, Hsu (1996)	1340 children (aged 8–12 years)	Wheeze
Peters et al. (1999)	3676 children	Wheeze
Spengler et al. (2004)	5951 children (aged 8–12 years)	Current wheeze
Strachan, Elton (1986)	165 children (aged 7–8 years)	Wheeze at age 0–5 years Wheeze at age 5–7 years Wheeze at age 0–5 years Wheeze at age 5–7 years
Venn et al. (2003)	416 children (aged 9–11 years); 193 with persistent wheeze and 223 controls	Wheeze

Dampness or mould measure	Risk estimate (95% CI)
Mould (minor damage)	1.2 (0.9–1.7)
Mould (major damage)	2.1 (1.2–3.6)
Mould (minor damage)	4.7 (2.1–10.5)
Mould (major damage)	6.0 (2.2–14.2)
Water leakage	1.15 (1.02–1.31)
Floor moisture	1.53 (1.25–1.87)
Visible dampness	1.53 (1.08–2.18)
Mould or dampness	
	1.00
	1.62 (1.22–2.15)
	1.65 (1.31–2.07)
	1.98 (1.47–2.66)
	1.00
	1.33 (0.98–1.82)
	1.56 (1.15–2.11)
	1.33 (0.84–2.10)
Self-reported dampness	1.36 (0.83–2.21)
Dampness	1.11 (0.63–1.93)
Mould	1.20 (0.73–1.99)
Stuffy odour	1.68 (1.03–2.74)
Water damage	1.43 (0.48–4.30)
Flooding	1.30 (0.69–2.45)
Water damage	1.15 ($p \geq 0.05$)
Mildew	1.94 ($p < 0.05$)
Water damage	1.53 (1.19–1.95)
Presence of mould	1.52 (1.19–1.94)
Damp	2.1^n ($p \geq 0.05$)
	1.7^n ($p \geq 0.05$)
Mould	2.2^n ($p \geq 0.05$)
	1.5^n ($p \geq 0.05$)
Living room damp:	
Very low	1.00
Low	1.37 (0.84–2.25)
Moderate	1.60 (0.73–3.49)
High	2.48 (0.90–6.82)
Kitchen damp:	
Very low	1.00
Low	1.14 (0.64–2.02)
Moderate	1.65 (0.77–3.55)
High	1.03 (0.33–3.16)

▶

Reference	Participants	Outcome
		Frequent nocturnal symptoms
		Frequent day-time symptoms
Yang et al. (1997b)[c]	4164 primary-school children (aged 6–12 years)	Wheeze
Yang et al. (1997a)[c]	4164 primary-school children (aged 6–12 years)	Wheeze
Yangzong et al. (2006)	2026 children (aged 12–14 years) living at altitudes > 3900 m	Wheeze at rest Wheeze after exercise Nocturnal wheeze Severe wheeze
Cuijpers et al. (1995)	470 primary-school children (aged 6–12 years)	Wheeze: boys Wheeze: girls

Dampness or mould measure	Risk estimate (95% CI)
Bedroom damp:	
Very low	1.00
Low	1.49 (0.94–2.36)
Moderate or high	1.26 (0.60–2.64)
Visible mould	5.10 (1.07–24.17)
Living room damp:	
Very low	1.00
Low	2.02 (0.81–5.04)
Moderate or high	3.86 (1.20–12.45)
Kitchen damp:	
Very low	1.00
Low	2.49 (0.90–6.89)
Moderate or high	3.56 (1.05–12.08)
Bedroom damp:	
Very low	1.00
Low	2.32 (1.04–5.16)
Moderate or high	7.03 (1.66–29.79)
Living room damp:	
Very low	1.00
Low	2.33 (0.93–5.83)
Moderate or high	3.23 (0.97–10.78)
Kitchen damp:	
Very low	1.00
Low	1.71 (0.59–4.96)
Moderate or high	1.37 (0.38–5.00)
Bedroom damp:	
Very low	1.00
Low	0.95 (0.42–4.96)
Moderate or high	1.72 (0.41–7.32)
Dampness in home	1.88 (1.36–2.59)
Dampness in home	1.81 (1.32–2.47)
Dampness problems	2.0 (1.1–3.6)
	1.3 (0.8–2.2)
	2.1 (1.1–4.1)
	2.3 (1.0–5.2)
Mould growth (always)	0.95 (0.16–5.46)
	2.69 (0.48–15.21)

▶

Reference	Participants	Outcome
		Wheeze: boys
		Wheeze: girls
		Wheeze: boys
		Wheeze: girls
Retrospective studies		
Alper et al. (2006)	858 primary-school children (aged 7 years)	No wheeze
		Wheeze in first 3 years
		Early transient wheeze
		Persistent wheeze
		Late-onset wheeze

Dyspnoea

Adults
Cross-sectional studies

Reference	Participants	Outcome
Nriagu et al. (1999)	693 adults	Shortness of breath with wheeze
Park et al. (2004)	323 employees in 13 college buildings	Shortness of breath
Brunekreef (1992)	3344 parents of children aged 6–12 years	Lower respiratory tract symptoms
Gunnbjörnsdottir et al. (2006)	15 995 adults (aged 20–44 years) who participated in the ECRHS	Nocturnal breathlessness
Skorge et al. (2005)	2401 adults (aged 26–82 years)	Dyspnoea grade 2
		Attacks of dyspnoea
		Dyspnoea grade 2
		Attacks of dyspnoea
		Dyspnoea grade 2
		Attacks of dyspnoea

Dampness or mould measure	Risk estimate (95% CI)
Mould growth (often)	0.46 (0.05–4.47)
	0.79 (0.06–10.66)
Mould growth (sometimes)	0.50 (0.13–1.89)
	0.54 (0.14–2.11)
Dampness and mould at home	1.0
	2.37 (1.52–3.69)
	2.28 (1.34–3.87)
	2.53 (1.30–4.87)
	2.46 (1.29-4.66)
Dampness at home	1.04 (0.46–2.34)
Water stains: continuous variable	1.7 (0.8–3.6)
Water stains: any	6.3 (0.8–51.1)
Any visible mould	2.6 (1.3–5.1)
Any mould odour	1.4 (0.7–3.2)
Any damp material or standing water	3.3 (0.9–11.9)
Factor combinations, weighted for water stains	2.7 (1.2–6.1)
Factor combinations, weighted for visible mould	2.5 (1.2–5.4)
Damp stains or mould	1.55 (1.27–1.89): women
	1.70 (1.38–2.09): men
Water damage	1.81 (1.50–2.19)
Wet floors	2.58 (1.93–3.45)
Visible moulds	1.72 (1.35–2.20)
Any dampness	1.80 (1.51–2.15)
Onset in damp homes	1.33 (1.09–1.63)
Remission in damp homes	0.68 (0.48–0.96)
Mould: only earlier	1.5 (0.92–2.47)
	1.7 (1.06–2.72)
Mould: earlier and last year	1.4 (0.91–2.10)
	1.1 (0.74–1.74)
Water damage: only earlier	1.4 (0.91–2.10)
	1.1 (0.74–1.74)

▶

Reference	Participants	Outcome
		Dyspnoea grade 2 Attacks of dyspnoea
		Dyspnoea grade 2 Attacks of dyspnoea
Haverinen et al. (2001)	1017 adults	Dyspnoea Nocturnal dyspnoea
		Dyspnoea Nocturnal dyspnoea
		Dyspnoea Nocturnal dyspnoea
		Dyspnoea Nocturnal dyspnoea
Gunnbjörnsdottir et al. (2003)	1853 young adults (aged 20–44 years)	Breathless when resting Breathless after effort Nocturnal breathlessness
		Breathless when resting Breathless after effort Nocturnal breathlessness
		Breathless when resting Breathless after effort Nocturnal breathlessness

Children
Cross-sectional studies

Reference	Participants	Outcome
Li, Hsu (1996)	1340 children (aged 8–12 years)	Shortness of breath
Cuijpers et al. (1995)	470 primary-school children (aged 6–12 years)	Shortness of breath: boys Attack of shortness of breath plus wheeze: boys
		Shortness of breath: boys Shortness of breath: girls

Dampness or mould measure	Risk estimate (95% CI)
Water damage: earlier and last year	1.2 (0.63–2.15)
	1.2 (0.65–2.07)
Mould	AF = 4.5 (1.3–7.5)
	AF = 4.1 (0.6–7.5)
Visible mould growth or odour at home *vs* neither	1.57 (0.94–2.63)
	2.02 (0.86–4.75)
Grade I[e]	1.00
	1.00
Grade II[e]	0.95 (0.49–1.85)
	2.22 (0.67–7.34)
Grade III[e]	1.78 (0.90–3.52)
	1.49 (0.49–4.57)
Mould only	0.90 (0.45–1.81)
	1.10 (0.64–1.88)
	0.94 (0.47–1.87)
Water damage only	1.15 (0.34–3.85)
	1.70 (0.70–4.16)
	0.75 (0.18–3.21)
Mould and water damage	3.24 (1.44–7.29)
	2.76 (1.36–5.60)
	1.00 (0.30–3.21)
Self-reported dampness	1.55 (1.01–2.38)
Dampness	1.49 (0.88–2.53)
Mould	1.55 (1.01–2.38)
Stuffy odour	1.59 (1.03–2.44)
Water damage	1.99 (0.82–4.83)
Flooding	1.16 (0.65–2.05)
Mould growth (always)	2.26 (0.54–9.49)
	1.23 (0.20–7.51)
Mould growth (often)	0.41 (0.04–3.76)
	1.93 (0.16–22.74)

▶

Reference	Participants	Outcome
		Shortness of breath: boys
		Shortness of breath: girls
		Attack of shortness of breath plus wheeze: boys
		Attack of shortness of breath plus wheeze: girls

Bronchitis

Children
Cross-sectional studies

Reference	Participants	Outcome
Yang et al. (1997b)[c]	4164 primary-school children (aged 6–12 years)	Bronchitis
Yang et al. (1997a)[c]	4164 primary-school children (aged 6–12 years)	Bronchitis
Peters et al. (1999)	3676 children	Bronchitis
Spengler et al. (2004)	5951 children (aged 8–12 years)	Current bronchitis
du Prel et al. (2006)	22 666 children (aged 6 years) in eastern Germany	Bronchitis, ever diagnosed
	6222 children (aged 6 years) in western Germany	Bronchitis, ever diagnosed
Li, Hsu (1996)	1340 children (aged 8–12 years)	Bronchitis

Other respiratory effects

Adults
Prospective studies

Reference	Participants	Outcome
Matheson et al. (2005)	845 adults (aged 20–45 years)	Bronchial hyperresponsiveness

Dampness or mould measure	Risk estimate (95% CI)
Mould growth (sometimes)	0.99 (0.32–3.01)
	0.81 (0.16–4.13)
	0.43 (0.09–2.07)
	0.44 (0.05–4.36)
Dampness at home	1.65 (1.28–2.14)
Dampness at home	1.58 (1.23–2.03)
Water damage	1.26 ($p \geq 0.05$)
Mildew	1.34 ($p < 0.05$)
Water damage	1.52 (1.14–2.03)
Presence of mould	1.70 (1.28–2.27)
Damp housing conditions	1.25 (1.13–1.37)
Damp housing conditions	1.30 (1.03–1.65)
Self-reported dampness	1.29 (0.96–1.73)
Dampness	1.89 (1.31–2.73)
Mould	1.89 (1.31–2.73)
Stuffy odour	1.40 (1.04–1.89)
Water damage	2.45 (1.24–4.82)
Flooding	1.17 (0.79–1.73)
Ergosterol[a]	0.90 (0.59–1.36)
Total fungi[a]	0.99 (0.77–1.27)
Other fungi[a]	0.91 (0.77–1.06)
Cladosporium[a]	1.0 (0.85–1.17)

TABLE A1.2. CONT.

Reference	Participants	Outcome
Retrospective studies		
Gunnbjörnsdottir et al. (2006)	15 995 adults (aged 20–44 years) who participated in the ECRHS	Nocturnal breathlessness
Cross-sectional studies		
Park et al. (2006)	888 occupants of a water-damaged building	Chest tightness Cough with phlegm
		Chest tightness Cough with phlegm
		Chest tightness Cough with phlegm
		Chest tightness Cough with phlegm
Lee et al. (2006)	24 784 adults (aged 26–50 years)	New-onset adult asthma
Children *Prospective studies*		
Dales et al. (2006)	332 children	Number of days with cough per year
Turyk et al. (2006)	61 children (aged 3–13 years) with asthma	Number of asthma symptoms
		Frequent asthma symptoms
		Number of asthma symptoms

Dampness or mould measure	Risk estimate (95% CI)
Water damage	1.81 (1.50–2.19)
Wet floors	2.58 (1.93–3.45)
Visible mould	1.72 (1.35–2.20)
Any dampness	1.80 (1.51–2.15)
Fungi [i]	1.8 (1.12–3.04)
	1.4 (0.82–2.30)
Fungi high, endotoxin low [j]	1.1 (0.46–2.69)
	1.2 (0.46–3.16)
Fungi low, endotoxin high [j]	1.3 (0.52–3.25)
	1.9 (0.73–5.00)
Fungi high, endotoxin high [j]	3.0 (1.42–6.32)
	2.7 (1.20–6.27)
Water damage	0.81 (0.50–1.25)
Visible mould	1.48 (1.07–2.01)
Endotoxin	$33.0 \pm 25.3°$
Penicillium in bedroom air:	
Tertile 1	1.0
Tertile 2	0.8 (0.2–2.8)
Tertile 3	3.8 (1.0–14.4)
	p for trend over tertiles = 0.09;
	p for linear trend = 0.06
Penicillium in bedroom air:	
Tertile 1	1.0
Tertile 2	1.2 (0.4–4.4)
Tertile 3	4.9 (1.2–20.2)
	p for trend over tertiles = 0.04;
	p for linear trend = 0.01
Total fungi in bedroom air:	
Tertile 1	1.0
Tertile 2	1.1 (0.3–3.7)
Tertile 3	1.1 (0.3–3.6)
	p for trend over tertiles = 0.92;
	p for linear trend = 0.48

▶

TABLE A1.2. CONT.

Reference	Participants	Outcome
		Frequent asthma symptoms
Retrospective studies		
Andriessen, Brunekreef, Roemer (1998)	1614 children with symptoms of asthma and chronic cough	Prevalence of lower respiratory tract symptoms Prevalence of phlegm
Cross-sectional studies		
Karevold et al. (2006)	3406 children (aged 10 years)	Tonsillopharyngitis
Nafstad et al. (2005)	942 children (aged 3–5 years) attending day-care centres	Nocturnal cough Heavy breathing or chest tightness
Dales, Burnett, Zwanenburg (1991)	14 799 parents of children aged 5–8 years	Lower respiratory tract symptoms Chronic respiratory disease

Allergy or atopy

Adults
Prospective studies

Reference	Participants	Outcome
Matheson et al. (2005)	845 adults (aged 20–45 years)	Atopy
Cross-sectional studies		
Dharmage et al. (2001)	485 participants in a follow-up study to the ECRHS	Risk for sensitization to fungi
Rennie et al. (2005)	1998 adults (aged 18–74 years)	Allergy
Norbäck et al. (1999)	455 adults; 98 prevalent cases of asthma and 357 controls	Increase in blood eosinophil concentration $\times 10^6$/l Increase in serum eosinophil cationic protein in µg/l Increase in blood eosinophil concentration $\times 10^6$/l Increase in serum eosinophil cationic protein in µg/l

Dampness or mould measure	Risk estimate (95% CI)
Total fungi in bedroom air:	
Tertile 1	1.0
Tertile 2	0.8 (0.2–2.8)
Tertile 3	1.3 (0.4–4.5)
	p for trend over tertiles = 0.71; p for linear trend = 0.16
Moisture stains	1.04 (0.88–1.24)
Mould	1.03 (0.84–1.26)
Moisture stains	1.05 (0.89–1.23)
Mould	1.06 (0.88–1.27)
Dampness at home	1.4 (1.1–1.6)
Dampness problems	1.23 (0.84–1.81)
	1.15 (0.64–2.07)
Dampness or mould	1.62 (1.48–1.78)
	1.45 (1.29–1.64)
Ergosterol[a]	1.38 (0.93–2.04)
Total fungi[a]	1.53 (1.00–2.32)
Other fungi[a]	1.17 (0.94–1.45)
Cladosporium[a]	1.05 (0.89–1.25)
Upper three quartiles *vs* first quartile:	
Ergosterol	Range: 2.4–2.7
Penicillium	Range: 0.5–0.8
Cladosporium	Range: 0.4–0.9
Damp housing	1.44 (0.84–2.45): men
	1.53 (1.05–2.24): women
Water damage or flooding	45 (11–79)
	1.0 (–1.2–3.2)
Dampness in the floor	27 (–25–79)
	–2.1 (–5.6–1.4)

▶

Reference	Participants	Outcome
		Increase in blood eosinophil concentration $\times 10^6$/l
		Increase in serum eosinophil cationic protein in µg/l
		Increase in blood eosinophil concentration $\times 10^6$/l
		Increase in serum eosinophil cationic protein in µg/l
		Increase in blood eosinophil concentration $\times 10^6$/l
		Increase in serum eosinophil cationic protein in µg/l
Schäfer et al. (1999)	1235 children	Skin-prick test reactivity to *Alternaria*
Spengler et al. (2004)	5951 children (aged 8–12 years)	Any allergy Respiratory allergy Any allergy Respiratory allergy
Jovanovic et al. (2004)	397 children: 199 with history of allergy 198 controls without	Serum IgE against fungi
du Prel et al. (2006)	22 666 children (aged 6 years) in eastern Germany 6222 children (aged 6 years) in western Germany	Allergy: ever diagnosed Allergy: ever diagnosed
Adults and children *Cross-sectional studies*		
Salo et al. (2006)	2456 adults and children	Diagnosed hay fever

Dampness or mould measure	Risk estimate (95% CI)
Visible mould on indoor surfaces	11 (–30–52)
	–0.9 (–3.6–1.8)
Mouldy odour	–45 (–7–97)
	–2.7 (–6.3–0.9)
At least one sign of building dampness	41 (2–60)
	0.5 (–0.4–3.4)
Dampness and visible mould	1.65 (0.69–3.93)
Water damage	1.26 (1.05–1.52)
	1.30 (0.95–1.77)
Presence of mould	1.51 (1.25–1.82)
	1.50 (1.11–2.02)
Measured mould	No association
Damp housing conditions	1.09 (0.93–1.28)
Damp housing conditions	1.20 (0.87–1.66)
Alternaria alternata concentration, adjusted model:	
1st tertile	1.00
2nd tertile	1.04 (0.71–1.51)
3rd tertile	0.92 (0.65–1.31)
Alternaria alternata concentration, adjusted model including other indoor allergens:	
1st tertile	1.00
2nd tertile	1.04 (0.71–1.53)
3rd tertile	0.91 (0.61–1.37)
Alternaria alternata concentration, adjusted model including other indoor allergens and dust weight:	
1st tertile	1.00
2nd tertile	1.03 (0.70–1.51)
3rd tertile	0.89 (0.59–1.35)

▶

Reference	Participants	Outcome
Children		
Prospective studies		
Müller et al. (2002)	475 premature infants and newborns at risk of atopy	Increased levels of specific IgE against grass
Douwes et al. (2006)	696 children with atopic mothers	Atopy at 4 years Atopy at 1 year
		Atopy at 4 years
Cho et al. (2006)	640 infants with at least one atopic parent	Positive skin-prick test to mould
		Positive skin-prick test to aeroallergens

Asthma, ever

Adults

Cross-sectional studies

Reference	Participants	Outcome
Nriagu et al. (1999)	693 adults	Asthma
Dales, Burnett, Zwanenburg (1991)	14 799 parents of children aged 5–8 years	Asthma
Skorge et al. (2005)	2401 adults (aged 26–82 years)	Asthma, ever

Children

Prospective studies

Reference	Participants	Outcome
Douwes et al. (2006)	696 children with atopic mothers	Doctor-diagnosed asthma

Dampness or mould measure	Risk estimate (95% CI)
Alternaria alternata concentration, adjusted model including other indoor allergens, dust weight and endotoxins:	
1st tertile	1.00
2nd tertile	1.07 (0.73–1.58)
3rd tertile	0.98 (0.64–1.51)
Aspergillus exposure > 100 CFU/m^3	5.28 (1.02–27.1)
Extracellular *Penicillim* or *Aspergillus* polysaccharides	0.40 (0.18–0.91) No association found (data not shown)
Extracellular *Penicillim* or *Aspergillus* polysaccharides, fungal glucan, endotoxins	No association found (data not shown)
Class of mould damage:	
None	RR = 1.0
Minor	RR = 1.6 (0.9–3.0)
Major	RR = 0.6 (0.1–4.0)
Class of mould damage:	
None	RR = 1.0
Minor	RR = 0.9 (0.6–1.2)
Major	RR = 1.6 (0.9–3.0)
Dampness at home	1.91 (0.61–6.01)
Dampness or mould	1.56 (1.25–1.95)
Mould: only earlier	1.4 (0.68–2.85)
Mould: earlier and last year	1.5 (0.69–3.47)
Water damage: only earlier	1.4 (0.78–2.62)
Water damage: earlier and last year	1.2 (0.49–2.85)
Glucan:	
Medium	0.63 (0.27–1.48)
High	0.70 (0.30–1.60)
Extracellular *Aspergillus* or *Penicillium* polysaccharides:	
Medium	0.78 (0.40–1.55)
High	0.42 (0.18–0.99)

TABLE A1.2. CONT.

Reference	Participants	Outcome
Ponsonby et al. (2000)	7241 children (aged 7 years)	Asthma
Cross-sectional studies		
Li, Hsu (1997)	46 children (aged 7–15 years)	Asthma
Lawson et al. (2005)	2038 schoolchildren in grades 1–6 in two communities	Asthma
Yang, Lin, Hwang (1998)	330 primary-school children (aged 6–12 years); 165 cases and 165 controls	Asthma

Asthma symptoms in people with asthma: intervention studies

Children
Prospective studies

Kercsmar et al. (2006)	62 symptomatic children with asthma (aged 2–17 years)	Acute care visits in 12-month follow-up period Proportion with ≥ 1 visit
		Average number of visits
		Acute care visits in 6-month post-remediation period Proportion with ≥ 1 visit
		Average number of visits
Bernstein et al. (2006)	19 mould-sensitized children with asthma (aged 5–17 years) living in houses with ventilation systems	Pulmonary function: difference in peak expiratory flow variability

Dampness or mould measure	Risk estimate (95% CI)
Mould observed by interviewer in child's bedroom	1.26 (0.87–1.81)
Mould reported by mother in home, excluding bathroom	1.20 (0.96–1.51)
Self-reported dampness	1.46 (0.55–3.85)
Mould	1.02 (0.39–2.69)
Water damage	0.70 (0.27–1.86)
Stuffy odour	3.19 (1.08–9.42)
Flooding	1.18 (0.27–5.17)
Dampness	1.01 (0.34–3.01)
Mould or dampness at home	1.54 (1.20–1.97)
Presence of a humidifier	1.08 (0.70–1.64)
Mould or dampness at home, first community	0.97 (0.53–1.79): boys
	0.64 (0.31–1.31): girls
Mould or dampness at home, second community	1.70 (0.98–2.94): boys
	1.76 (1.01–3.07): girls
Dampness at home	2.65 (1.52–4.62)
Thorough remediation of indoor dampness and mould	
	17.2% *vs* 36.4% in controls ($p = 0.15$)
	0.28 *vs* 0.91 in controls ($p = 0.06$)
	3.5% *vs* 33.3% in controls ($p = 0.003$)
	0.07 *vs* 0.52 in controls ($p = 0.004$)
Ultraviolet radiation to reduce microbial exposures over 2 weeks	−0.068 ($p = 0.03$)

▶

TABLE A1.2. CONT.

Reference	Participants	Outcome
		Pulmonary function: difference in FEV_1 Difference in wheeze severity score Difference in shortness of breath severity score Difference in chest tightness severity score Difference in cough severity score Difference in number of days with wheeze Difference in number of days with shortness of breath Difference in number of days with chest tightness Difference in number of days with cough Difference in medication use (number of inhalations)

Asthma symptoms in people with asthma: observational studies

Children
Prospective study

Reference	Participants	Outcome
Wever-Hess et al. (2000)	Children (aged 0–4 years) with newly suspected asthma (doctor-diagnosed)	Exacerbation Recurrent exacerbation

Cross-sectional studies

Reference	Participants	Outcome
Bonner et al. (2006)	149 children (aged 3–5 years) with asthma	Number of hospitalizations in previous 12 months Number of episodes of wheeze in previous 12 months Number of nights awake in previous 2 weeks
Forsberg et al. (1997)	15 962 children (aged 6–12 years)	Asthma attacks
Sotir, Yeatts, Shy (2003)	128 568 middle-school children	Upper respiratory tract infection-triggered wheeze with asthma risk factor among children reporting current wheeze

Dampness or mould measure	Risk estimate (95% CI)
	−0.87 (*p* = 0.32)
	−0.02 (*p* = 0.4)
	−0.22 (*p* = 0.04)
	−0.3 (*p* = 0.04)
	−0.28 (*p* = 0.26)
	−0.25 (*p* = 0.24)
	−2.75 (*p* = 0.02)
	−3.50 (*p* = 0.04)
	−2.00 (*p* = 0.28)
	−38 (*p* = 0.04)

Damp housing	7.6 (2.0–28.6)
	3.8 (1.1–12.8)

Moisture or mildew	
	3.31 (1.62–6.75)
	3.25 (1.8–6.0)
	2.19 (1.40–3.41)
Moisture stains or mould: current exposure	1.2 (0.9–1.5)
Moisture stains or mould: during child's first 2 years	1.6 (1.3–2.1)
Mould or mildew in house	Prevalence odds ratio = 1.72 (1.48–2.01)

Reference	Participants	Outcome

Altered lung function

Adults
Prospective studies

Dharmage et al. (2002)	35 young adults with current asthma and sensitization to fungi in the ECRHS	Peak flow variability

Cross-sectional studies

Gunnbjörnsdóttir et al. (2003)	1853 young adults (aged 20–44 years)	FEV_1 (ml) FVC (ml) FEV_1 (ml) FVC (ml) FEV_1 (ml) FVC (ml)
Norbäck et al. (1999)	455 adults; 98 prevalent cases of asthma and 357 controls	Percentage predicted FEV_1 Average PEF variability

Ebbehøj et al. (2005)	522 teachers in 15 public schools: 8 water damaged and 7 undamaged	Male teachers
		  FEV_1
		
		  FVC
		
		  KCO
		
		  DLCO
		
		Female teachers
		  FEV_1
		
		  FVC
		
		  KCO
		
		  DLCO

Dampness or mould measure	Risk estimate (95% CI)/Test result
Visible mould	1.4-fold increase ($p \leq 0.02$)
Mould only	−36 (−103–32)
	−16 (−98–65)
Water damage only	−77 (−207–54)
	29 (−129–186)
Mould and water damage	−20 (−141–102)
	−85 (−231–61)
No sign of dampness	108% (SD, 16%)
Dampness in the floor	102% (SD, 13%) ($p < 0.05$)
No sign of dampness	3.8% (SD, 3.1%)
Dampness in the floor	5.4% (SD, 5.0%) ($p < 0.01$)
Total estimated dose of mould:	
Low	101.0 (10.6)
Medium	95.4 (16.1), NS
High	99.9 (19.2), NS
Low	105.8 (14.2)
Medium	101.0 (19.5), NS
High	103.0 (19.1), NS
Low	116.0 (16.6)
Medium	119.6 (19.4), NS
High	117.7 (14.7), NS
Low	107.1 (15.5)
Medium	103.3 (18.4), NS
High	105.6 (10.8), NS
Low	105.6 (12.3)
Medium	103.5 (13.9), NS
High	105.8 (12.7), NS
Low	111.7 (20.0)
Medium	106.5 (15.3), NS
High	108.5 (12.7), NS
Low	105.6 (14.0)
Medium	106.9 (15.3), NS
High	107.5 (17.3), NS
Low	97.0 (13.3)
Medium	94.7 (13.9), NS
High	97.6 (14.7), NS

TABLE A1.2. CONT.

Reference	Participants	Outcome
Children *Prospective studies*		
Bernstein et al. (2006)	19 mould-sensitized children with asthma (aged 5–17 years) living in houses with ventilation systems	Peak flow variability, difference between placebo and active conditions FEV_1 (l/s), difference between placebo and active conditions
Brunekreef et al. (1989)	4625 children (aged 8–12 years)	FVC FEV_1 FEV_{25-75} FVC FEV_1 FEV_{25-75} FVC FEV_1 FEV_{25-75} FVC FEV_1 FEV_{25-75}
Cross-sectional studies		

Douwes et al. (2000)	148 children (aged 7–11 years) of whom 50% had self- or parent-reported chronic respiratory symptoms	Peak flow change per increase of two geometric SDs in exposure:
		    Non-symptomatic ($n = 64$)
		
		    Symptomatic ($n = 72$)
		
		    Asthmatic ($n = 34$)

Strachan et al. (1990)	1000 children (7 years old)	Reduction in FEV_1:
		    > 10%
		    ≤ 10%
		Reduction in FEV_1:
		    > 10%
		    ≤ 10%
		Reduction in FEV_1:
		    > 10%
		    ≤ 10%
		Reduction in FEV_1:
		    > 10%
		    ≤ 10%
		Reduction in FEV_1:
		    > 10%
		    ≤10%

Dampness or mould measure	Risk estimate (95% CI)/Test result
Ultraviolet radiation to reduce microbial exposure	−0.068 ($p = 0.03$)
	−0.87 ($p = 0.32$)
Mould	0.44[p] (−0.27–1.15)
	0.03 [p] (−0.75–0.82)
	−1.62 [p] (−3.19 – −0.02)
Water damage	0.25 [p] (−0.61–1.12)
	0.35 [p] (−0.59–1.30)
	0.46 [p] (−1.49–2.45)
Basement water	0.16 [p] (−0.54–0.87)
	−0.14 [p] (−0.92–0.65)
	−1.14 [p] (−2.74–0.44)
Dampness	−0.09 [p] (−0.75–0.58)
	−0.21[p] (−0.93–0.52)
	−1.06 [p] (−2.55–0.44)
(1→3) β-D-glucan	
	0.94-fold decrease (0.75–1.18)
	1.33-fold decrease (1.06–1.67)
	1.45-fold decrease (1.10–1.92)
Airborne mould in living room	381 CFU/m^3
	282 CFU/m^3
Airborne mould in child's bedroom	285 CFU/m^3
	206 CFU/m^3
Airborne mould in other room	407 CFU/m^3
	278 CFU/m^3
Pooled samples, total	354 CFU/m^3
	253 CFU/m^3
Pooled samples, *Penicillium* spp.	62 CFU/m^3
	49 CFU/m^3

▶

Reference	Participants	Outcome

		Reduction in FEV_1:
		  > 10%
		  ≤ 10%
		Reduction in FEV_1:
		  > 10%
		  ≤ 10%
		Reduction in FEV_1:
		  > 10%
		  ≤ 10%
		Reduction in FEV_1:
		  > 10%
		  ≤ 10%

Retrospective studies

Reference	Participants	Outcome

Andriessen, Brunekreef, Roemer, 1998)	1614 children with symptoms of asthma and chronic cough	Mean daily variation in PEF
		  Per CV: morning
		  Per CV: evening
		  Per minimum morning variation
		
		Mean daily variation in PEF
		  Per CV: morning
		  Per CV: evening
		  Per minimum morning variation

Dampness or mould measure	Risk estimate (95% CI)/Test result
Pooled samples, *Cladosporium* spp.	12 CFU/m^3 13 CFU/m^3
Pooled samples, *Sistotrema brinkmanii*	3.1 CFU/m^3 3.8 CFU/m^3
Pooled samples, white rot basidiomycetes	1.0 CFU/m^3 1.7 CFU/m^3
Pooled samples, *Mycelia sterilia*	1.0 CFU/m^3 0.7 CFU/m^3
Moisture stains	0.98 (0.92–1.03)[q] 0.98 (0.92–1.04)[q] 1.01 (0.95–1.07)[q] 0.99 (0.97–1.02)[q]
Mould	1.05 (0.98–1.12)[q] 1.04 (0.97–1.11)[q] 1.04 (0.97–1.11)[q] 1.00 (0.97–1.03)[q]

Abbreviations and footnotes

AF   attributable fraction;
CFU   colony-forming units;
CI   confidence interval;
CV   coefficient of variation;
DLCO   total lung diffusion capacity for carbon monoxide;
ECRHS   European Community Respiratory Health Survey;
FVC   forced vital capacity;
FEV1   forced expiratory volume in 1 second;
FEV25-75 forced expiratory flow between 25% and 75% of FVC;
IRR   incidence rate ratio;
KCO   alveolar diffusion constant for carbon monoxide ;
PEF   peak expiratory flow;
NS   not significant;
RR   relative risk .

[a] The effect of doubling allergen or fungal exposure on the risk for of developing new clinical outcomes.

[b] Stark et al. (2003) defined lower respiratory tract infection from answers to the question: "Since we last spoke on (date given), has your child had pneumonia, croup, bronchitis, or bronchiolitis diagnosed by a doctor?" The primary outcome variable was at least one report of lower respiratory tract infection in the first year of life.

[c] These publications cover the same populations, and the risk estimates reported are based on identical analyses with slightly different odds ratios.

[d] As this relates to absence of dampness, it implies that dampness at home is a risk factor for asthma.

[e] Grade I, no visible moisture damage, minor moisture damage, one patch of deteriorated interior finish or covering; grade II, single observation of a damaged interior structural component, single patch of deteriorated interior finish or covering, as in grade I, plus other damage of same or lower severity; grade III, presence of a damaged interior structural component, as in grade II, with other damage of the same or lower severity; or functional element that required partial or total renewal, with or without other damage.

[f] Adjusted for association between personal exposure to particles and microbial aerosol and symptom diary responses.

[g] Adjusted for association between microenvironmental concentrations of particles and microbial aerosol at home and symptom diary responses.

[h] Adjusted for association between microenvironmental concentrations of particles and microbial aerosol at work and symptom diary responses.

[i] No interaction models.

[j] Interaction models.

[k] Full variate model.

[l] Multivariate model omitting any lower respiratory infection in year 1.

[m] Multivariate model omitting dust-borne *Aureobasidium*.

[n] Relative odds of morbidity.

[o] Incidence (mean ± standard deviation).

[p] Difference in mean pulmonary function, expressed as a percentage of the grand mean, between children living in damp houses and children living in dry houses.

[q] Adjusted mean daily variation in PEF over the study period; daily variation = (morning – evening PEF)/((morning + evening PEF)/2)) (in %).

Annex 2.
Summary of in vitro
and in vivo studies

Table A2.1. Summary of in vitro studies on the effects of exposure to microbes or their isolates, including studies relevant to microbial exposures in damp buildings

Cell type	Exposure
Studies on the effects of bacteria or fungi	
Human alveolar epithelial cells	Spores of *Streptomyces anulatus*
Mouse macrophages, human macrophages, human alveolar epithelial cells	Spores or cells of *Mycobacterium avium, Mycobacterium terrae, Aspergillus versicolor, Penicillium spinulosum, Stachybotrys chartarum, Bacillus cereus, Pseudomonas fluorescen, Streptomyces californicus*
Mouse macrophages	*S. anulatus* grown on different building materials
Mouse macrophages	Fungal spores of *S. chartarum, A. versicolor, P. spinulosum* and spores of *S. californicus* grown on wetted plasterboard
Mouse macrophages	Live and heat-killed fungal spores of *Aspergillus fumigatus*
Studies on the effects of mycotoxins and other microbial products	
Mouse macrophages	Mycotoxin-extractions of *S. chartarum* spp. isolated from mouldy buildings
Human PBMC	Pure toxins: citrinin, gliotoxin, patulin
Human, mouse and rat neural cell lines	Pure toxin: fumonisin B_1
Human monocytes	Pure toxins: citrinin, gliotoxin
Hamster lung fibroplasts, monkey kidney cells, primary rat kidney cells	Pure toxin: ochratoxin A
Mouse primary cortical neuronal cultures	Nigerlysin, haemolysin produced by *Aspergillus niger*

Main findings	Reference
Induction of cytotoxicity and inflammatory responses (NO, IL-6)	Jussila et al. (1999)
All tested bacteria induced inflammatory responses (IL-6, TNF-α, NO) in mouse macrophages, but only *S. californicus* and environmental mycobacteria provoked inflammation (NO, IL-6) in human cells. Inflammatory potential of the tested fungi was weak. Human cells were more resistant to cytotoxicity than mouse cells.	Huttunen et al. (2001, 2003)
The most intense cytotoxic and inflammatory responses (NO, TNF-α, IL-6) were induced by spores grown on plasterboard.	Roponen et al. (2001)
The brand, composition and liner and core materials of plasterboard affected the inflammatory responses (NO, IL-1β, IL-6 and TNF-α) and cytotoxicity induced by the spores. Incomplete prevention of microbial growth by biocides increased the toxicity of spores of *S. chartarum*.	Murtoniemi et al. (2001b, 2002, 2003)
mRNA expression of TNF-α, MIP-1α, MIP-1β, and MCP-1 after exposure to live, but not to heat-killed spores	Pylkkänen et al. (2004)
Isolates of the satratoxin-producing chemotype were highly cytotoxic. Atranone-producing chemotypes induced inflammatory responses, unlike the pure atranones B and D.	Nielsen et al. (2002)
Mycotoxins inhibited IFN-γ-producing T cells.	Wichmann, Herbarth, Lehmann (2002)
Increased production of ROS in mouse and rat cells; decreased GSH levels; increased lipid peroxidation and necrotic cell death in all cell lines	Stockmann-Juvala et al. (2004)
Inhibition of anti-inflammatory IL-10 and relative overproduction of pro-inflammatory IL-6 and TNF-α	Johannessen, Nilsen, Lovik (2005)
Induction of apoptosis and oxidative DNA damage in cell lines and primary cells	Kamp et al. (2005)
Rapid loss of cell viability	Donohue et al. (2006)

TABLE A2.1. CONT.

Cell type	Exposure
Human, mouse and rat cell lines of neural and glial origin	Pure toxin: fumonisin B_1
Mouse alveolar macrophages	Spore-extracted toxins of *S. chartarum*
Human alveolar epithelial cells	Pure toxins: citrinin, gliotoxin and lipopolysaccharides

Studies on interactions between microbes and microbial products

Cell type	Exposure
Mouse macrophages	Spores of *S. californicus* with spores or cells of separately grown *A. versicolor*, *P. spinulosum*, *S. chartarum*, *B. cereus*, *M. terrae*, and *P. fluorescens* or various toxins of *S. chartarum*
Mouse macrophages	Combinations of *S. californicus, S. chartarum, A. versicolor* and *P. Spinulosum* co-cultivated on wetted plasterboards
Mouse macrophages	Spores of co-cultivated *S. californicus* and *S. chartarum* and known cytostatic agents produced by streptomycetes
Mouse macrophages	Amoebae plus spores of *S. californicus* or *Penicillium spinolosum*

Main findings	Reference
Caspase-3 activity increased in all cell lines, except human cells of neural origin; glial cells were more sensitive.	Stockmann-Juvala et al. (2006)
Toxins induced cytotoxicity, apoptosis, DNA damage and p53 activation.	Wang, Yadav (2006)
Reduced intracellular antioxidant GSH and TGF-β1 levels at low mycotoxin concentrations	Johannessen, Nilsen, Lovik (2007)
Synergistic increase in IL-6 production only when macrophages were concomitantly exposed to *S. chartarum* and *S. californicus*. Of the toxins of *S. chartarum* tested, trichodermin and 7-α-hydroxytrichodermol produced a similar synergistic response with *S. californicus*.	Huttunen et al. (2004)
Co-cultivation of *S. chartarum* and *A. versicolor* synergistically increased the cytotoxicity of the spores.	Murtoniemi et al. (2005)
Microbial interactions during co-cultivation potentiated the ability of the spores to induce apoptosis, cell cycle arrest, DNA damage, p53 accumulation and cytotoxicity in macrophages. The cytostatic agents tested induced similar responses, but not the spores of separately grown microbes.	Penttinen et al. (2005b, 2006, 2007)
Amoebae potentiated the cytotoxic and inflammatory (NO, IL-6, TNF-α) properties of the microbial spores.	Yli-Pirilä et al. (2007)

Table A2.2. In vivo studies on the effects induced by exposure of the airways to microbes relevant to exposure in damp buildings (past 10 years)

Animal (exposure route)	Exposure
Mouse (nasal)	*Stachybotrys atra (chartarum)* (two strains)
Mouse (nasal), repeated dosing	*Stachybotrys atra (chartarum)* (two strains)
Rat (intratracheal)	*S. chartarum*
Rat (intratracheal)	*S. chartarum* (methanol-treated and untreated spores)
Juvenile mouse (intratracheal)	*S. chartarum, Cladosporium cladosporioides* and iso-satratoxin F
Mouse (intratracheal)	*S. californicus*
Rat pups (intratracheal)	*S. chartarum*
Mouse (aspiration)	*S. chartarum* (extract)

Main findings	Reference
Strain-specific effects. Spores containing satratoxin caused intra-alveolar and intestinal inflammation with haemorrhagic exudate in alveolar lumina. They also caused necrotic changes and milder inflammation after exposure to spores without satratoxin.	Nikulin et al. (1996)
Toxic and non-toxic spores. Decreased platelet count, increased leukocytes, erythrocytes, haemoglobin and haematocrit; inflammatory changes were more severe in the lungs of mice receiving toxic spores. No histopathological changes were seen in the thymus, spleen or intestines *Toxic spores.* Dose-dependent severe inflammatory changes occured in bronchioles and alveoli. Haemorrhage occured in the alveoli	Nikulin et al. (1997)
Cytotoxicity and inflammation with haemorrhage; increase in albumin, LDH, haemoglobin, macrophages, polymorphonuclear leukocytes, eosinophils and lymphocytes in BALF in a time-dependent manner; loss of body weight	Rao, Brain, Burge (2000)
Increases in albumin, LDH, haemoglobin and polymorphonuclear leukocytes in BALF after exposure to untreated spores; loss of body weight. Methanol-extracted spores had no significant effects – that is, adverse effects related to methanol-soluble toxins in spores.	Rao, Burge, Brain (2000)
Altered surfactant metabolism in *S. chartarum*-treated mice (increased conversion from heavier alveolar surfactant H to the lighter surfactant L, elevated phospholipid concentration in surfactant H)	Mason et al. (2001)
BALF and serum. Increased levels of IL-6, TNF-α, total protein, albumin, haemoglobin and LDH in BALF and increased expression of iNOS in BAL cells *Histopathology.* Mild-to-moderate inflammation in lung	Jussila et al. (2001)
BALF. Increased numbers of macrophages, lymphocytes, neutrophils and pro-inflammatory cytokines (IL-1, TNF-α) *Histology.* Fresh haemorrhage, sparse haemosiderin-laden macrophages, and thickened alveolar septa infiltrated by lymphocytes and mononuclear cells	Yike et al. (2002)
BALF. Increased total protein, LDH, total cell number, lymphocytes, neutrophilia, eosinophilia *Serum and BALF.* Elevated total IgE	Viana et al. (2002)

TABLE A2.2. CONT.

Animal (exposure route)	Exposure
Mouse (intratracheal)	*P. spinulosum*
Mouse (intratracheal)	*M. terrae*
Mouse (intratracheal)	*A. versicolor*
Mouse (intratracheal)	*S. chartarum* (two strains: high and low stachylysin producers)
Mouse (intratracheal)	*S. chartarum*, *C. cladosporioides* and iso-satratoxin F
Mouse (intratracheal), repeated dosing	*S. californicus*
Mouse (nasal)	*S. chartarum*, satratoxin producing and non-producing strains

Main findings	Reference
BALF. Transiently elevated IL-6 and TNF-α, and neutrophils	Jussila et al. (2002b)
Histopathology. Mild, transient inflammation in lung	
Sustained biphasic inflammation in lungs; bacteria remain up to 28 days in lungs.	Jussila et al. (2002a)
First phase (6 h to 3 days). Increased IL-6 and TNF-α, neutrophils, total protein, albumin and LDH in BALF	
Second phase (7–28 days). Increased TNF-α, iNOS in BAL cells, total protein, albumin and LDH in BALF; monocytes and lymphocytes in airways.	
Histopathology. Mild-to-moderate inflammation in lungs	
BALF. Transient increase in IL-6 and TNF-α, neutrophils, macrophages and lymphocytes; elevated total protein, albumin, haemoglobin and LDH after exposure to high dose	Jussila et al. (2002c)
Histopathology. Elevated neutrophils in alveoli and bronchiolar lumen; transient hyperaemia and pale patches in lung necroscopy	
Both strains. Granulomatous inflammatory reaction	Gregory et al. (2003)
High stachylysin-producing strain. More stachylysin in lung tissue and macrophages than with low stachylysin-producing strain	
S. chartarum and *C. cladosporioides.* Increased granuloma formation in lung; depression of alveolar space	Rand et al. (2003)
S. chartarum. Alveolar accumulation of erythrocytes; dilated capillaries; elevated haemosiderin; reduced collagen IV distribution in lung granulomas	
Iso-satratoxin F. No inflammatory response in lungs	
Immunostimulation in lungs and systemic immunotoxicity (spleen)	Jussila et al. (2003)
BALF. Increased total protein, albumin, LDH, IL-6, TNF-α, neutrophils and macrophages; increased numbers of activated and unactivated CD3⁻ CD4⁻ T lymphocytes and unconventional CD3⁻ CD4⁻ lymphocytes in lung tissue	
Histopathology. Decreased cell numbers in spleen, increased numbers of neutrophils and mononuclear cells in alveoli and in bronchiolar lumen; no signs of genotoxicity in leukocytes	
Both strains. Increase in BALF monocytes, neutrophils and lymphocytes and lung mRNA levels of pro-inflammatory cytokines and chemokines	Leino et al. (2003)
Satratoxin-producing strain. Higher mRNA levels of chemokine CXCL5/LIX	

TABLE A2.2. CONT.

Animal (exposure route)	Exposure
Mouse (intratracheal)	*S. chartarum*, trichothecene (JS58-17)- and atranone (JS58-06)-producing strains; *C. cladosporioides*
Infant rats (intratracheal)	*S. chartarum* (intact, autoclaved and ethanol-extracted spores)
Mouse (aspiration)	*Penicillium chrysogenum*
Mouse (nasal)	Satratoxin G isolated from *S. chartarum*
Mouse (nasal)	*S. chartarum* plus ovalbumin sensitization
Rat (intratracheal)	*S. chartarum*
Mouse (intratracheal)	Atranones A and C from *S. chartarum*
C3H7Hej mouse, BALB/c mouse, C57BL76j mouse (intratracheal)	*S. chartarum*

Main findings	Reference
BALF. Total protein, albumin, pro-inflammatory cytokine (IL-1, TNF-α) and LDH responses significantly different (time and dose dependently) by fungal species (*S. chartarum vs C. cladosporioides*) and fungal strain *(JS58-17 vs S58-06)* Low doses of both of *S. chartarum* strains caused significantly higher responses than *C. cladosporioides.*	Flemming, Hudson, Rand (2004)
Reduced alveolar space (largest effect with intact spores) Potency of different spore preparations on inflammatory cells, cytokine and protein concentrations: intact > autoclaved > extracted	Yike, Rand, Dearborn (2005)
Allergic asthma-like responses with repeated dosing (dose dependently). Immediate respiratory responses and metacholine hyperresponsiveness and increased BALF eosinophils, IL-5, total IgE and serum total IgE	Chung et al. (2005)
Elevated expression of proapoptotic genes in olfactory sensory neurons and epithelium Cumulative effects with low doses on five consecutive days Elevated mRNA expession of pro-inflammatory cytokines and chemokines in nasal airways and adjacent olfactory bulb of the brain (neurotoxicity)	Islam, Harkema, Pestka (2006)
Effects of sensitization: Increased eosinophils and neutrophils Granulomatous inflammatory infiltrates in lungs, increased mRNA levels of proinflammatory cytokines IL-1 and TNF-α and a chemokine (CCL3/MIP-1 α) Down-regulated airway hyperresponsiveness and decrease in Th2 cytokines	Leino et al. (2006)
Decreased alveolar macrophage viability, increased lysosomal enzyme cathepsin D activity	Pieckova et al. (2006)
Elevated macrophages, neutrophils, MIP-1, TNF-α, IL-6 in BALF	Rand et al. (2006)
Mouse strain differences affected responses to *S. chartarum* BALB/c only strain to show significant increase in BAL cytokines (KC, MCP-1, MCP-3, MIP-1 α, MIP-1β, MIP-γ, MIP-2, CCL-5, IL-1α, , IL-1β, IL-3, IL-6, IL-18, leukaemia inhibitory factor, macrophage colony factor and TNF-α)	Rosenblum Lichtenstein et al. (2006)

Animal (exposure route)	Exposure
Mouse (nasal)	Roridin A (macrocyclic trichothecene)
Rat pups (intratracheal)	*S. chartarum*: high (JS58-17) and low (JS58-06) trichothecene-producing strains

Main findings	Reference
Apoptosis in olfactory sensory neurons	Islam et al. (2007)
Upregulated mRNA expression of proapoptotic gene *Fas* and pro-inflammatory cytokines in ethmoid turbinates	
Simultaneous exposure to lipopolysaccharides magnified roridin A-induced apoptosis and inflammation in the nasal tract	
High trichothecene-producing strain. Lower proteolytic activity	Yike, Rand, Dearborn (2007)
Both strains.	
Increased neutrophils, IL-1β and TNF-α	
Reduced collagen IV labelling in spore-induced lung granulomas	

Abbreviations

BAL	bronchoalveolar lavage;
BALF	bronchoalveolar lavage fluid;
CCL	chemokine ligand;
GSH	glutathione;
IFN-γ	interferon-γ;
Ig	immunoglobulin;
IL	interleukin;
iNOS	inducible nitric oxide synthase;
KC	keratinocyte-derived chemokine;
LDH	lactate dehydrogenase;
MCP	monocyte chemoattractant protein;
MIP-1	macrophage inflammatory protein 1;
NO	nitric oxide;
PBMC	peripheral blood mononuclear cells;
ROS	reactive oxygen species;
Th2	T-helper 2 cytokines
TGF	transforming growth factor;
TNF-α	tumour necrosis factor alpha